FROM
BREAST CANCER
TO
Blessed Answer

One Woman's Journey
from Diagnosis to Tattoos

ADRIA HOWARD-MOORE

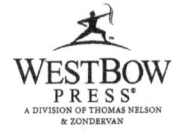
WESTBOW
PRESS®
A DIVISION OF THOMAS NELSON
& ZONDERVAN

Copyright © 2021 Adria Howard-Moore.

All rights reserved. No part of this book may be used or reproduced by any means, graphic, electronic, or mechanical, including photocopying, recording, taping or by any information storage retrieval system without the written permission of the author except in the case of brief quotations embodied in critical articles and reviews.

This book is a work of non-fiction. Unless otherwise noted, the author and the publisher make no explicit guarantees as to the accuracy of the information contained in this book and in some cases, names of people and places have been altered to protect their privacy.

WestBow Press books may be ordered through booksellers or by contacting:

WestBow Press
A Division of Thomas Nelson & Zondervan
1663 Liberty Drive
Bloomington, IN 47403
www.westbowpress.com
844-714-3454

Because of the dynamic nature of the Internet, any web addresses or links contained in this book may have changed since publication and may no longer be valid. The views expressed in this work are solely those of the author and do not necessarily reflect the views of the publisher, and the publisher hereby disclaims any responsibility for them.

Any people depicted in stock imagery provided by Getty Images are models, and such images are being used for illustrative purposes only.
Certain stock imagery © Getty Images.

Unless otherwise indicated, all Scripture taken from the New King James Version®. Copyright © 1982 by Thomas Nelson. Used by permission. All rights reserved.

Scripture quotations marked (NIV) are taken from the Holy Bible, New International Version®, NIV®. Copyright © 1973, 1978, 1984, 2011 by Biblica, Inc.® Used by permission of Zondervan. All rights reserved worldwide. www.zondervan.com The "NIV" and "New International Version" are trademarks registered in the United States Patent and Trademark Office by Biblica, Inc.®

ISBN: 978-1-6642-3756-8 (sc)
ISBN: 978-1-6642-3757-5 (hc)
ISBN: 978-1-6642-3755-1 (e)

Library of Congress Control Number: 2021912265

Print information available on the last page.

WestBow Press rev. date: 07/22/2021

To Mom

Thank you for pointing me to Jesus.

INTRODUCTION

IF YOU WANT TO KNOW WHAT AN ELEPHANT IS, YOU MUST DO MORE THAN TOUCH ITS TRUNK

My mother always told me I was special, and when I was a kid, I believed I was special. In society, however, I was just another person—nothing extraordinary. Like many kids, I was picked on in school. You know how it is; children can be very mean. The high school I attended was rough. How rough was it? I had to abstain from drinking anything during the day, for instance, because I couldn't use the bathroom. Certain groups of girls had claimed the ladies' john as their territory, and if you tried to use one, you could get seriously hurt. It was difficult for me to understand because I wasn't raised with that mentality. I was taught that you loved everyone. I could have fought back, but I was instructed to turn the other cheek. All the negative comments made about me and to me during my school years solidified in my mind that I wasn't special.

I attended art school and had a hard time there too. I have a natural talent for drawing and painting, but my low self-esteem never allowed me to stretch myself and explore my creativity. If I got a negative comment about my artwork, it just confirmed my feelings that it was no good, and I just gave up. My attic contains many unfinished works.

I tried being involved in what I thought were *true* churches.

One ended up being a cult and the other was very legalistic. Let me explain what I mean. The word *legalism* isn't in the Bible. This term describes a doctrine that emphasizes rules and regulations by which one attains and keeps one's salvation. In essence, it's up to the individual's works. As we know, every one of us makes mistakes, and this "faith" system made me feel like a real failure. I should have known better; no matter how good I tried to be, my works were *not* going to get me anywhere. Sooner or later, I *was* going to mess up. Isaiah 64:6 says, "But we are all like an unclean thing, And all our righteousnesses are like filthy rags; We all fade as a leaf, And our iniquities, like the wind, Have taken us away."

The Bible asserts that our good deeds, on which many rely to get brownie points with God, are like filthy rags to Him. The term *filthy rags* doesn't mean the week-old laundry that's sitting in your hamper or the soiled cloth a car mechanic uses to wipe his hands. It's actually very disgusting, as it comes from the Hebrew word *iddah*,[1] which means the bodily fluids from a woman's menstrual cycle. Therefore, our greatest efforts at being holy are as repulsive to God as a used feminine hygiene product. Pretty gross, huh? We are commanded to do good, but these good deeds are *not* what gets us into paradise. C. S. Lewis, author of *The Lion, the Witch, and the Wardrobe*, explains it like this: "The Christian does not think God will love us because we are good, but that God will make us good because He loves us."

Over the years, two failed marriages wreaked havoc on my already-battered ego. Being a believer, I always had faith that I was worth *something*, but I didn't think it was much. Because of my fear of being put down and wanting to be a part of the crowd, I wasn't a strong and faithful Christian.

Eventually, I was blessed to start attending a Bible-believing church that had a true heart for God. Yes, I get that no matter where

---

[1] "H5708 - 'iddah - Strong's Hebrew Lexicon (KJV)." Blue Letter Bible. Accessed Jan. 16, 2021, https://www.blueletterbible.org//lang/lexicon/lexicon.cfm?Strongs=h5708&t=kjv.

you go, there are problems. Charles H. Spurgeon, theologian and preacher, once cautioned people against joining a perfect church: "The day we find the perfect church, it becomes imperfect the moment we join it."

I must have a hard head because it's taken me years to finally just *begin* to get it. I'm not saying I have arrived; no, on the contrary, I'm saying my eyes are finally opening to the truth, strength, and reality of God. I am learning, day by day, about the magnificent power and wonder of the Almighty. The more I learn about the character of God, the more I marvel that He should even consider me. We read in Psalm 8:4, "What is man that You are mindful of him, And the son of man that You visit him?"

Yet He does, and I have experienced this in an intimate and personal way. It's not a cookie-cutter pattern that is a one-size-fits-all blueprint for all of humanity. Christian radio host and author Nancy DeMoss Wolgemuth hit the nail on the head when she said, "God masterfully orchestrates and weaves together every detail of our lives in jaw-dropping ways."

I guess that's what separates true Christianity from religion. Many people say they are spiritual, but *spiritual* can have a very broad definition. In my experience, most people I know who say this really mean, "I believe in God, but I want to worship Him in the way *I want to. I* make the rules." In other words, they are their own god. They want to live life on their own terms but still feel good about it in relation to an almighty Creator. I also have a sneaking suspicion they don't want to be beholding to any organized religion.

There are others who pick and choose from any number of religions, kind of like an à la carte religious buffet menu, going down the line and selecting what they like from each one. Reminiscent of the hippies' license of the 1960s—"If it feels good, do it." I'm not sure that some really delve into what God Himself wants from us. A lot has to do with their feelings.

God is vast and deep. My husband kids me when I say, "God is so smart," but He really is! He is so much more than we give

Him credit for. Some reject God based on what they think and don't bother to get to know Him before deciding to write Him off. They make up their own version of who they *think* God is. Again, I wholeheartedly agree with C. S. Lewis, when he said, "I want God, not my idea of God."

There is a parable found in Buddhist, Jain, and Hindu texts about some blind men who each describe an unusual creature—an elephant. It goes something like this:

> A group of blind men heard that a strange animal had been brought into town. None of these men had any idea what an elephant was so knew nothing about it. Out of curiosity, they all decided to go investigate. When they found the creature, each began to touch it to learn about this animal. The first man, who was holding the elephant's trunk, said it was like a snake. However, another man, who had his hands on the beast's large ears, disagreed and said it seemed like a kind of fan. The man who was inspecting its tusk declared he thought it was like a smooth spear. The blind man who placed his hands on the elephant's side was sure the animal was more like a strong wall. Finally, the fifth man felt its tail and described it like a rope.

People use this parable to say there are different ways of looking at something, and people can have their *own truths*. What I see in this story, however, is each man attempting to know what this creature was. They each experienced a specific characteristic of the elephant but erroneously assumed that what they had felt was *all there was* to this creature. Sometimes, we do the same thing with God. We see something about God (or perhaps something we *think* is attributed to God) and assume that is all there is to Him. If we turn to the scriptures, Jeremiah 29:13 reads, "And you will seek Me and find Me, when you search for Me with all your heart."

In my mind, if these blind men had really wanted to know what the elephant was all about, they would have continued using all the senses they had to learn about this creature. Instead, in some versions of this parable, they suspect each other of lying and come to blows with one another.

God *wants* us to get to know Him. *Really know Him.* So much so that He came down to earth to be one of us. He knows what it's like to hurt, to be rejected, to be lonely. He isn't just a parable. He is a real person, documented by witnesses and historians.[2]

One of my favorite Christmas songs is "How Many Kings," sung by Downhere. This song asks:

> 'Cause how many kings stepped down from their thrones?
> How many lords have abandoned their homes?
> How many greats have become the least for me?
> And how many Gods have poured out their hearts
> To romance a world that is torn all apart?
> How many Fathers gave up their Sons for me?

He reached down to us. He didn't spare His own beloved Son because we are so important to Him. From where I sit, religions are a way for man to connect and reconcile to God; true Christianity, however, is God's way to connect and reconcile with us. We can't do it. Remember the filthy rags?

The words contained in the following chapters are what I have learned about this magnificent Creator of ours and how He used cancer to show me that I am special to Him.

---

[2] Lawrence Mykytiuk, "Did Jesus Exist? Searching for Evidence Beyond the Bible," *Biblical Archaeology Review* (January/February 2015): 45–51, https://www.biblicalarchaeology.org/daily/people-cultures-in-the-bible/jesus-historical-jesus/did-jesus-exist.

Chapter 1
A GIFT?

Life was going well. It was simple and happy. I was in good shape, didn't tire easily, had lost a few pounds, and felt great—better than I had my whole life. My job was quite physical, and it wasn't unusual for me to walk at least five miles each day, in addition to lifting, climbing, and carrying heavy objects. I love the morning, so waking up at three forty-five to go to work was not a problem. There was only one thing. My left breast began to hurt every now and then. It was getting worse as time went on. I checked for a lump, but I couldn't feel anything. Still, it didn't look right. There was a strange dimpling near my nipple that hadn't been there before, and I thought something was wrong.

This wasn't anything I wanted to deal with right then. Tim and I were planning a vacation to celebrate our sixth wedding anniversary. We were taking a cruise to the Bahamas with another couple. Well, not just another couple. My best friend of forty-two years, Rosa, and her sweetheart, Keir! This would be great. Seven days and six nights of enjoying the sun, relaxing poolside, and doing many other things that we'd never done before, such as swimming with dolphins. I was so excited. I couldn't just ruin everyone's vacation by going to the doctor now. It would have to wait until we got back.

And it was a wonderful vacation. We had excellent weather and ate and ate and ate! We sampled everything from ice cream cones to caviar. We saw Broadway-style shows, enjoyed the hot tub, and played pool, which is quite challenging when the ship lists and the balls go hither and yon. All in all, it was a blast!

I tried not thinking about having to go to the doctor when we got home, but it was in the back of my mind the whole time. For instance, when we arrived in Nassau and donned our wet suits, making us look a little like misshapen seals, I thought about something I had seen on a talk show years earlier. A woman had gone swimming with dolphins, as we were doing, and once in the water, a dolphin stayed near her and even bumped her. The dolphin trainer asked the woman if she was dying; if the dolphin swim was one of her last wishes. She said no and gave the same answer when he asked if she had cancer. After her return home, she saw a doctor, who found a tumor in one of her lungs. Somehow, the dolphin knew. I wondered if a dolphin would be able to detect cancer in me. It turned out that one of the little rascals did bump me on my left shoulder—and hard! I told myself it was just because I was in the wrong place at the wrong time.

After we got home, I put off contacting the doctor for about a week but knew I had to act and forced myself to call. I remember reluctantly dialing the phone to get an appointment for an exam so I could get a mammogram. My appointment was for that Saturday morning. *Great!*

I really dislike going to doctors, dentists, therapists, psychologists—any *ists*—and today was no exception. I am a patient of a medical office where multiple doctors hang their shingles, and patients see whichever physician is available at the time. That day, I was assigned a dedicated female doctor. I could tell Dr. Toller was committed to her profession by the way she sat with me. (This is not her real name. I've chosen to use pseudonyms for each of the medical professionals who treated me.) There was no rushing through so she could get to her next appointment, finish her day, and maybe sneak in a round of golf. She took her time and asked a lot of questions. When the tone of her voice changed, I could tell that there was a chance something was bad.

No lump could be felt, but she was not at all happy about the strange dimpling on my left breast. She scolded me for not being diligent about my health. Although my sister had gotten breast cancer a decade earlier, I had neglected to get regular checkups. She contacted a nearby radiology center and arranged for me to go for a mammogram. She stressed to them that I was to have it done *today*, saying, "You *will* make time for this patient." She didn't care how they had to rearrange appointments to squeeze me in, just that they do it *now*. Gulp!

After the appointment with Dr. Toller, I met up with Rosa for breakfast. We were chatting about our fabulous trip and sharing photos. Eventually, I told her where I had been and that the doctor had scheduled me for a mammogram later in the day. I could see the fear in Rosa's face. Maybe it wasn't fear; maybe it was concern, but the way she looked at me made me worry. She even offered to go with me. I said no and tried to brush it off like it was no big deal.

I told her I'd be fine, but now I wasn't so sure. Reality was hitting me. Had I known all that is involved in the treatment of cancer, I probably would have been terrified. Ignorance, as they say, is bliss.

I was uneasy going to the radiology center. I suppose most women who go there are scared half to death. I was trying not to have that mindset. The facility wasn't a cold, sterile, or impersonal environment. I felt more like I was at a spa than a radiology facility. They had me disrobe in a changing room and offered me a warm cloth (not paper) robe to wear. The waiting room was decorated in soft colors and had upholstered chairs. Next to me was a bowl of chocolate candy on a bookcase that held mostly magazines and a

Bible. I picked up a magazine to pass the time because I didn't want to pick up the Bible and admit that I was afraid.

A nurse stuck her head in to make sure I was OK and told me I would be seen shortly. I suppose they didn't want me sitting there with my thoughts for too long. I looked at the bookcase again, and this time I picked up the Bible. I guess that was the point when I acknowledged there was a problem, and I needed God's assurance.

When I went into the room where the mammography machine was, I was pleasantly surprised. The room was dimly lit, and the machine itself had a soft white glow. The light slowly changed colors, adding a soothing ambiance to the room. Soft music played in the background, and pictures of butterflies were on the walls. The nurse who performed the procedure was sweet and explained everything that was going to be done. She apologized in advance for the discomfort I was about to experience and talked to me the entire time to keep my mind occupied.

After the mammogram, I was back in the robe in the waiting room. I prayed. I don't exactly remember what I prayed, but I think I asked God to help me trust Him, no matter the outcome. When I spoke to the nurse again, she said she couldn't give me the results of the test but that it didn't look good. She wanted me to be prepared for bad news.

Now it was time to have an ultrasound. Again, the technician was very polite, and I appreciated how she paid attention to the little details to ensure I was comfortable, like heating up the gel that was applied to my breasts before the ultrasound. They took great strides to make sure my experience was as pleasant as it could be, considering the circumstances.

After both tests, the nurse told me that I needed a biopsy, and she could make the appointment for me if I liked. (Well, no, I didn't like, but I *had* to.)

When I returned home, it was difficult to tell Tim. I tried to be brave as I said the words *cancer* and *biopsy*. Poor Tim. When I told him, all the blood just streamed out of his face. This affected me deeply, as I didn't want to hurt my loved ones. Next, I contacted my two older daughters, Erin and Alyson. When I told them, they took it well, and I felt encouraged after speaking with them. Next, I called my two sisters, and that too was fine, but then I spoke with my cousin, whom I shall call Rupert. All I can say is after that phone call, I felt miserable. Even though some of the things Rupert said may have been true, it cut me to the quick to hear him say it so harshly. He seemed angry. It had been hard enough to call each of these people I loved to tell them the grim news; I didn't want someone jabbing their finger in my face, telling me all the things I *should* have done to prevent this. I realize now that everyone responds to bad news differently. I just wasn't prepared for it at that moment.

Negative verbal responses are difficult, but so are body language responses. I'll explain. Tim was scheduled to play his drums for church that Sunday. Prior to each service (there are four), the musicians and singers all gather in a circle and pray. Tim requested prayer for me, not specifying the need. Later, however, as he was quietly telling one of his friends what was going on, one of the ladies overheard their conversation. During the worship service while she was singing, she made eye contact with me, and I got the most pitiful look imaginable. It made me feel uncomfortable. I realized she was empathizing with me, but I didn't like that *look*. I was trying to avoid thinking about it (cancer), and I most definitely didn't want people to feel sorry for me. Since then, I have learned that I can't control how others respond. However, I can (usually) control how I respond.

The radiology center scheduled my biopsy for Wednesday at 11:00 a.m. at a nearby hospital. I was nervous but peaceful. It's hard to explain being peaceful when you're facing this, except to quote Philippians 4:7—"and the peace of God, which surpasses all understanding, will guard your hearts and minds through Christ Jesus."

God took care of me throughout this whole ordeal in intimate and personal ways. I marvel now as I look back at it all. The first time I was aware of God's active participation in this journey was when we walked into the hospital for the biopsy. God sent someone to comfort us. Listen to me when I say this: never underestimate your work for God. If He asks you to do something or sends you somewhere, and you question what good it will do, just trust Him and *do it*! You might think it's a nothing-burger, but God sees the whole picture. He knows all the tiny details.

The Christian missionary Paul, in his letter to the Corinthian church, wrote in 1 Corinthians 15:58, "Therefore, my beloved brethren, be steadfast, immovable, always abounding in the work of the Lord, knowing that your labor is not in vain in the Lord." I reiterate the last part of this verse: "knowing that your labor is not in vain in the Lord." Can we say that about anything else?

We entered the hospital's waiting room and signed in at the information desk. The receptionist directed us where to go wait—and what do you know? My dear friend Nancy was there. Nancy and I have spent many a Sunday sitting side by side behind the consoles at church, controlling the lighting effects and projecting the worship songs out to the congregation. It turns out that a mutual friend of ours was also at the hospital for a same-day procedure, and Nancy was supporting her. God had given Nancy a twofer that day! It was no coincidence that both of us were at the same hospital at the same time. I emphasize here that I do not believe in coincidences. God is sovereign.

> Let the heavens rejoice, and let the earth be glad;
> And let them say among the nations, "The Lord reigns." (1 Chronicles 16:31)
>
> But our God is in heaven; He does whatever He pleases. (Psalm 115:3)

A third party may read this and think that the events I treasure are not a big deal. However, in my world they are. They're specific to me, personally. When I consider that it was the Almighty's hand in all of this, I marvel. It sounds a bit strange, but I think God used cancer to show me that He loves me, that I'm forgiven, and that I can rest in Him.

Now, back to the hospital: I thought, *How wonderful of God to provide a prayer warrior for us.* Just seeing her there comforted me. We talked and laughed, and I knew she was praying, and that was the greatest gift she could have given me that day.

The room where they performed the biopsy was small and quite packed with the five of us: the doctor, the technician, a nurse, Tim, and me. Tim had to sit in a chair in the corner, and the nurse stood to my right and held my hand. She explained exactly what would happen and what I would hear. When the doctor came in (who just happened to be Dr. Toller's husband), he reiterated what the nurse had told me. He said he'd be inserting a hollow needle to take out pieces of breast tissue from the suspicious area and that I'd hear a click when it clamped down on the tissue. I would hear it twice since there were two masses. I had another mammo performed right before the doctor saw me, so he knew exactly where to direct the needle. He then told me he would insert metal markers to indicate where the masses were. This way, when I had future mammograms, they would know where to look. He said the only way I'd get rid of the markers was if I had surgery, and they removed the area. They used to tattoo a dot on your breast to indicate where the lump or mass was, but I guess they found markers to be more precise. Then, using his professional doctor voice, he told me something that wasn't easy to hear: "I am so positive there's cancer that if this test comes back negative, I'm going to do it again."

I went numb.

Then he went to work, injecting me with two local anesthetics—*ouch*. And the clicks they told me about seemed much louder than I anticipated. Maybe it was because the small room was so quiet, and the sound echoed off the walls. Oh, and did I mention that the good doctor then squished down on my already sore breast after he removed the needle so the area didn't bleed? *Double ouch.* I was drained and exhausted. A month ago, I was fine; I was in the Caribbean, enjoying the sun and surf, but now I was here in the hospital, afraid and in pain. However, in the midst of it all, God gave me peace. In the deafening stillness of the little room, I tried to whisk myself away and fill my mind with a Bible verse about peace—but I couldn't think of any. Rather than concentrate on the reality of what was happening, I kept thinking, over and over, *peace, peace, peace*, and God graciously provided it. His peace enabled me to be calm and handle this stark reality. Pretty cool.

I thought I was done when the doctor put down his instruments, but no. Another mammogram awaited me. *Really?* I thought. *Do they even know how done I am with this right now?* Then they bandaged me up and sent me home. Silly me; I went to work the next day with an ice pack tucked in my brassiere. Naturally, I wound up going home early and needed to take the next day off as well. I was in more pain than I'd expected. I only told one coworker that I'd had a biopsy. I can't explain it, but I felt very vulnerable. The people around me who saw me, day in and day out, didn't know what was going on, and I wanted it that way.

I realized that to deal with cancer, I needed peace. I didn't want to be a panicky mess. Personally, I think I can endure just about anything if I'm calm and have the assurance that *God's got this.*

Joni Eareckson Tada, author and artist, who tragically became a quadriplegic while only a teenager, said it this way during an interview with *Tabletalk* magazine—and I concur wholeheartedly:

> Deuteronomy 31:6, where God tells me, "Be strong and courageous. Do not be afraid or terrified [of quadriplegia, chronic pain, or cancer], for the Lord your God goes with you; he will never leave you nor forsake you." I'm convinced a believer can endure any amount of suffering as long as he's convinced that God is with him in it. And we have the Man

of Sorrows, the most God-forsaken man who ever lived, so that, in turn, He might say to us, "I will never leave you; I will never forsake you." God wrote the book on suffering and He called it Jesus. This means God understands. He knows. He's with me.[3]

I looked up the word *peace* and found that the Hebrew word *shalom* doesn't just mean peace, as we understand peace. It means wholeness, completeness, soundness, health, safety, and prosperity and implies that it's permanent, not fleeting. When we read Isaiah 26:3—"You will keep him in perfect peace, Whose mind is stayed on You, Because he trusts in You"—the word translated as "perfect" is also the Hebrew word shalom. Therefore, a literal interpretation of "perfect peace" is shalom, shalom—peace, peace. That's multiplied peace! This verse shows us that peace is given to those who trust in the Lord. Was this cancer a gift to teach me things that I would not be able to learn any other way? When one thinks about gifts one would like to receive, I'm quite positive cancer is not on the list. However, Proverbs 25:4 shows how going through something painful can turn into something beautiful: "Take away the dross from silver, And it will go to the silversmith for jewelry."

Silver must be purified before it can be used. It is heated in fire, and as it melts, the dross, or impurities, rise to the surface, and the silversmith skims it off. The silver is heated again, this time at a higher temperature, which brings more dross to the surface to be removed. It's only after this purifying process that the silversmith can turn the precious metal into something useful and beautiful. It didn't sound pleasant, but I was so optimistic. I figured God was

---

[3] Joni Eareckson Tada, "A Purpose in the Pain: An Interview with Joni Eareckson Tada," October 1, 2011, https://www.ligonier.org/learn/articles/a-purpose-in-the-pain-an-interview-with-joni-eareckson-tada.

going to purify me to use me to do something wonderful. After all, I reasoned, "I'm strong! I can do this!"

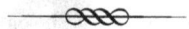

I thought I would get the results sooner than my appointment a week later, since the Drs. Toller were married. I imagined them discussing my case over their morning coffee (like they had nothing better to talk about). I hate waiting. Patience is not one of my strongest attributes. Not knowing is worse than knowing in my book. My imagination is vivid. I'd rather have a straight-on, in-your-face reality than a hurry-up-and-wait situation. As it turned out, I played quite a few waiting games during this journey. After what the doctor said to me, I expected a cancer diagnosis, but I wanted all the details.

Eventually, I did get a call from the radiology center, but of course they wouldn't discuss anything with me over the telephone. They preferred to have a face-to-face consultation, which makes sense. I didn't want to go, but, like I said, I was so optimistic at this time that I wasn't afraid. Tim and I drove the thirty minutes to the center, and we were happy and upbeat. Tim didn't let on that he was nervous, but I knew he was. We signed in and soon got called into one of the offices. The decor in the office was warm and homey. I got the feeling I was in someone's reading room, rather than a medical facility. The nurse came in and gazed at me with the *look*. (*Sigh*) and softly said, "You have cancer." She then proceeded to tell me a lot of other information, which I don't think I even heard. I wanted to say to her, "Can we cut to the chase? I want this *out of me*! Let's get this done." I had no idea how long this process would be and how it would try my patience again and again.

She told me I needed a surgeon, and she highly recommended Dr. Nett. What did I know about surgeons? I had no idea how to go about selecting the medical personnel who would be treating me for years to come. If I was given a choice of two oncological surgeons, I might have flipped a coin to decide. Since his office was close, and this nurse thought he was well qualified, this was a no-brainer, and I went with him.

She left the office to make the appointment with the surgeon, and while she was gone, I made a joke to Tim about our next *Star Trek* convention. We've drummed up some outrageous cosplay (short for costume play) outfits that have earned us prizes and some recognition from the *Star Trek* alumni themselves. For instance, we wound up on Robert Picardo's Twitter feed (he played the Doctor in *Star Trek: Voyager*) and on Adam Nimoy's website. Adam is Leonard (Spock) Nimoy's son. He wanted a picture with us because he felt we were honoring his father. This might not sound like much, but to us, it made the many hours creating these getups all worth it. Rosa, Tim, and I have been Talosians, Vulcans, hologram characters, and several assorted aliens from the imagination of Gene Roddenberry. But I digress.

"I guess for our next convention, I can be Ilia," I blurted out. She was a character from *Star Trek: The Motion Picture*—a bald female character. I remember thinking what an awful, awful joke that was and how inappropriate too. Tim gave me a look that told me that statement made him quite uncomfortable, and he wasn't sure if he should laugh or not.

The nurse returned to the room and said that my appointment was the following day. I don't remember much after that, except I felt like everything bad that could happen *would* happen. I figured I would have a mastectomy, chemo, and radiation and wind up looking like the *Toxic Avenger* (a campy, B-horror movie, filmed in New Jersey, where a mild-mannered boy falls into a vat of toxic waste and becomes an unlikely and very disfigured superhero). In my mind, the prognosis was bleak.

Tim willingly and lovingly jumped into the arduous task of being the caretaker and had the unenviable job of relaying the news to everyone. I didn't want to repeat the news over and over, answering the same questions again and again. I knew I had to let

Rosa know, but I couldn't bear to tell my best friend in all the world that I was going to be the Toxic Avenger. She was at work, and I knew the news would trouble her. I didn't want her to drive home upset. So, I called Keir. I poured out my heart to him and begged him to please, *please* wait to tell her in person. Then, I instructed him to show her a picture of Lieutenant Ilia, thinking it might add a bit of levity to the bad report. Well, in true Keir fashion, he got it all wrong and called her at work. Rosa, of course, didn't know what was going on, and Tim had to untangle the convoluted tale she had been told.

Tim took his role as caregiver very seriously. He's a fixer. This was his way of coping and being able to *do* something. He doesn't like to feel helpless. As soon as we walked in the door, he dutifully called a list of people to tell them I had cancer and what was planned for the next few days. Rupert gave Tim a rough time, and their conversation got heated. This added stress that neither Tim nor I needed or wanted. I didn't understand why Rupert reacted the way he did. Tim was doing the best he could, and we were keeping people informed as timely as we could. We were overwhelmed and frightened. Then the thought crossed my mind that the news might have scared Rupert too.

I got up for work and didn't have much of an appetite. By day's end, I was exhausted, both mentally and physically. While going through this transition from *normal* to cancer patient, it was hard to think straight. I had so many emotions all raging at once. I wanted to be angry, and Rupert seemed like a good candidate to receive that anger. Dr. Nett, however, pointed out that not everyone handles bad news in the same way. He said I needed to show patience to others. That was very wise advice.

Two weeks had passed since I found out I had breast cancer. During those fourteen days, my brain was preoccupied with what had just happened and wondering what was next. I received so much love from my dear, sweet husband, my wonderful children, my Rosa, my sisters, and the few friends in whom I confided. I felt such peace, but as the band Boston sang, "It's more than a feeling." I didn't know this, but throughout this entire journey, I would be hearing from God and sensing His will. He was teaching me to hear His voice.

The Bible says in Psalm 37:4, "Delight yourself also in the Lord, And He shall give you the desires of your heart." If someone asks you what the desire of your heart is, you might say it's healthy kids, a hefty bank account, or extended lifespan—but cancer? No, cancer wasn't a gift. The more I thought about this, I realized that cancer was just the conduit through which God was drawing me closer to Him. He was using a very ugly thing to create something beautiful. I envisioned a dark, long, winding, hilly road along which God wanted me to walk. I had a strong sense that I *wasn't* going to die from this disease. I could also see the end of this road, and it was open and bright, like the sun was shining. I had assurance that He would be with me the entire time. *That*, indeed, was a great gift.

In Isaiah 61, there is a phrase "give them beauty for ashes." In the time this was written, it was typical for people to sit in or cover themselves with ashes to express loss or mourning. Isaiah 61 is a prophetic chapter, foretelling God's plan for Israel and the arrival of the Messiah. He planned to deliver Israel, heal the brokenhearted, comfort those who mourned, and free the captives. I can look at these verses, millennia after they were written, and receive encouragement and hope. I know He will make a trade with me and give me *beauty for ashes*. I can trade in my pain and suffering for something wonderful that is beyond my imagination. I figured whatever lay ahead, if I was in God's will, that was the absolute best place to be. I knew something big was looming over the horizon. Whatever it was, I need not fear because I knew "my Redeemer lives"![4]

---

[4] Job 19:25.

Chapter 2

THE LORD OF PEACE

During this journey, I had to make countless decisions. Believe me when I say it got to the point where I didn't even want to choose what to eat for dinner. It is tempting to just go with the flow or to delegate that job to my caregiver, but I knew I should do neither.

It is easier to let your caregivers handle the brunt of everything and make all the decisions, but it's not fair to them. Caregivers get drained and irritated and probably feel like heels if they complain. Yes, we are the ones who are physically sick, but we should always consider how much the caregivers suffer right along with us. They too do not need any added stress.

I knew it was my body, and I had to live with the results. If there were problems down the line, I didn't want to have resentment or remorse for not taking the reins myself. I learned early on to pray about any choices I had to make—"If any of you lacks wisdom, let him ask of God, who gives to all liberally and without reproach, and it will be given to him" (James 1:5)—do research, seek advice from professionals and others—"Listen to counsel and receive instruction, That you may be wise in your latter days" (Proverbs 19:20)—and then come to my conclusion. It wasn't until midway through my treatment, after watching a video on four women's journeys through breast cancer, that I realized many women base their course of treatment on their feelings or emotions. That shocked me. Emotions can be overwhelmingly strong but are not a sure foundation on which to base vital decisions. I was also grateful that God was protecting me from the terror that many people feel when they face this awful disease. I became keenly aware and thankful that God was protecting and guiding me. I was *not* alone in this. Yes, Tim was with me, but in the dark of night, when it was just me and my brain and reality came crashing down on me like a ton of bricks, there is One who was always there.

> "Have I not commanded you? Be strong and of good courage; do not be afraid, nor be dismayed, for the Lord your God *is* with you wherever you go." (Joshua 1:9)

Some people are great decision-makers. Me? I'm always second-guessing myself. Then I look back at what I chose and play the "shoulda, woulda, coulda" song in my head. For this journey, though, the choices I had to make would affect me for the rest of my life. I couldn't be flippant about them. As I mentioned earlier, I came up with a kind of formula that enabled me to be more confident about my selections (listen, learn, pray, decide).

However, you also need to know *when* to stop researching and stop asking, as too much information can put your brain into overload. It will leave you frustrated and confused.

Furthermore, I came to realize that sometimes the options given to me weren't the only ones I had. Indeed, I considered how it would affect my family and finances. In the long run, though, I knew that regardless of what others thought, *I* had to live with the outcomes. And money? Well, that comes and goes (mostly goes). I needed to be secure enough with my selection that no matter what, I was satisfied with the result. It's a rough row to hoe.

Whether you ask for it or not, you will get advice. There are those who offer it out of concern and love; I can deal with that. I think it's wonderful that they care, and I know they are doing it from a loving place. Then there are people who think there are only two opinions—theirs and the wrong one. Some may come across like that but aren't being arrogant; they are just so satisfied with their results. It's a "this worked for me, so it *must* work for you" kind of thing. I came upon all these types. A few expressed their thoughts about where I was going to go for treatment. They gave their opinions about various hospitals that were more prestigious. I knew they just wanted me to get the best care. Then there were others who would insist I go to a certain hospital, or see a specific doctor, and when I didn't, they were incredulous. I found the best way for me to handle the last type was to smile, say thank you, and avoid discussing it with them ever again.

I received one piece of advice that I didn't have to think long and hard about. An individual suggested I post *everything* on social media. When I heard this, the hairs on the back of my neck stood up. For this person, it had been a blessing. She had received so much encouragement from all the friends she had online that it helped her tremendously. She delighted in the advice and comfort that came her way. Personally, I felt that was *not* a practice I should adopt. I didn't want to open up and blab to the whole world, "Hey, everybody! I have breast cancer." I could just see it now. I would be getting the *look* electronically—no, thanks.

Choosing the medical network that would treat me was critical. Since I live relatively close to both Philadelphia and New York City, there were many options open to me. On the other hand, I didn't want to add the financial burden of traveling too far every time I needed treatment. I had to consider that I had a forty-hours-a-week job with limited time off, and I couldn't fathom taking a two-or three-hour road trip (one way) every couple of weeks. The medical bills would start to mount, and I wanted to avoid any added expenses. The trip in and out of Manhattan alone could ring up a bill of at least two hundred dollars each visit. Besides, our local hospital was now part of a larger network of hospitals in New Jersey that had access to many specialists in this field. I thought it prudent to stick close to home. My particular brand of cancer wasn't advanced, had not spread, and was run-of-the-mill, so to speak. I didn't see the need to use a Howitzer when a pistol would do.

The decision to use Dr. Nett as my surgical oncologist was an excellent one. When I met him, it was uncanny to me how closely he resembled my pastor. (I was a little uneasy having my breasts examined by Pastor Gregory Pauschal's doppelganger!) Their mannerisms and demeanors were so similar that I wouldn't have been surprised to hear they were related. Dr. Nett was younger than Pastor Greg. If I had to guess, I'd say in his early fifties. His tall stature was complemented by his perfect posture and slender frame. He looked me right in the eyes when he spoke to me, heard what I had to say, and answered my questions without rushing me. Although he had most likely had these same conversations with a thousand other women, he spoke to me as if I was his first patient. He was thorough, thoughtful, confident, knowledgeable, and to the point. He didn't beat around the bush. That's my kind of doctor. In the immortal words of Han Solo, "I prefer a straight fight to all this sneaking around." I want to know up front what I'm dealing with.

Dr. Nett said he didn't feel a lump. (Dr. Toller had said the same thing.) The masses were near my nipple on my left breast. He was not pleased that, due to insurance regulations, he had not been able to examine me before the biopsy. His voice was calm and confident, and he intimated that I might be able to get away with *just* a lumpectomy and the removal of some lymph nodes. (Yay! No Toxic Avenger!)

He wanted me to meet with an oncologist and recommended Dr. Dawn, whose office was just around the corner. He warned that she was an excellent doctor but short on bedside manner. I guess this was information he had received secondhand from other patients because I found her to be caring and concerned. She also had quite a sense of humor.

Then he told me something that sent shivers down my spine. He wanted me to go for an MRI. He didn't realize to whom he was telling this, but I guess he could see the look of panic on my face.

"It won't be a problem," he said. "Have a drink before you go."

"Uh-uh! I'll throw up," I protested.

"OK, I'll give you Valium," he said, undaunted.

Two Valium later, I found myself back at the radiology center for a "quickie" MRI. It seemed that once again, insurance companies dictated processes that didn't make much sense. I had to have a quick in-and-out MRI at the center before I went to the hospital to have the *real* MRI. When I went into the room where the machine was, I froze. I was shaking and felt like I was going to lose my lunch and mess my pants. It was only a fifteen-second in-and-out, but it terrified me. How would I go through the *actual* MRI? I'm pretty sure many of the patients in the waiting room were alarmed and wondered what had just happened when, after the scan, I frantically rushed out of the building, nearly in tears.

Let me explain. I suffer from claustrophobia. I don't do elevators—not ever. Before all this, Tim had never seen me in an elevator. Rosa has yet to ride an elevator with me. I'm certain none of my children has ever seen me in an elevator. I have walked up twenty-four flights of stairs—in heels—rather than get in an elevator. I break out in a cold sweat going *near* an elevator. I get the creeps when I go into a bank and see the vault open. I panic if the zipper in my dress gets stuck, and I can't get out of it. When I say I'm claustrophobic, I mean it. This is not just something that makes me feel uncomfortable. No, it's an irrational, unexplainable, paralyzing fear. This fear is debilitating, overwhelming, and terrifying.

Tim waited in the car for me while I ran in to have the scan. When I came out, he was shocked at what he saw. I was crying and shaking and absolutely petrified. I was trying to communicate to him just how frightened I was, but he didn't get it. We prayed, and Tim kept telling me to breathe because I was hyperventilating. I don't remember the ride to the hospital, but when we got there, I remember fumbling with my cell phone, trying to look up scripture verses for comfort. I was also a little annoyed because Tim seemed a million miles away. *He doesn't understand*, I thought. *Not in the least.* In his defense, how can you explain something to someone when it doesn't even make sense to you?

A young man came into the waiting room and told me I was next. He saw that I was a wreck and probably knew this wasn't going to be easy. He directed me to the changing room; it had lockers for your belongings while you were being scanned. Each locker had a key hanging on a keychain in the shape of a pink boxing glove. I got it. We're women, and we have to fight, but I really began to hate the color pink. I was trying very hard to be brave. I've heard it said that you don't know how brave and strong you are until you have breast cancer. Well, I thought I was, but in reality, I'm a big chicken.

The nice technician called me in to the room where the monster of a machine was. I looked at the MRI as if it were a giant beast, waiting to have me for its next meal. I was shaking. The nice technician and I went back and forth a few times about how this procedure needed to be done.

First, the technician: "It's only thirty minutes; not bad."

"*Says you!*" I disputed.

"You know you need to have this done," he returned calmly.

I felt resigned to this fate. "Yes, I know."

He sighed. I could tell he was getting frustrated with me. It was the end of the day, and I was probably his last patient. So many thoughts raced through my head. Panicking, I thought, *OK, I've got to do this. I can't do this, but God can. I'm so scared. Trust God. I have to go to the bathroom. What if I lose it and go potty in the machine?*

God was tearing down the strongholds in my life and I needed to trust Him. I was so scared, and I knew I had to put feet to my faith and trust God. But how? What does faith look like? It's easy to say you believe in God, but to honestly put all you've got into trusting Him in a life-or-death situation; that's hard. To me, this *was* a life-or-death situation. I think I would have preferred a firing squad over this MRI. I was adamant, however, that I was not going to leave the hospital without doing this. There was no way I was going to make a second trip back here. I took a deep breath and followed the nice but exasperated technician's directions; I lay facedown on a flat bed. I thought it was neat that it had breast-shaped convex forms, so I wasn't uncomfortable lying on my stomach. The technician was very discreet when opening my gown. He had it down to a science and never once was I unrobed in front of him. That said, I'm very certain there are other things he would rather have seen than a hysterical, middle-aged woman's cancerous breast.

Tim was allowed in the room at this point, and he stood by my feet. The nice technician explained he would pull me into the machine and insert an IV into my arm. At that point, he would start the machine. He told me it was extremely noisy but that I must lie still. He then tried to put a set of sound-canceling headphones on me, and I nearly jumped off the bed. The heavy headset made me feel even more caged in. I tried not to panic. Wanting to protect my ears, the patient technician suggested I use earplugs.

This was really going to happen. As I was slowly moved into the machine, I tried to think about how God was with me. My arms were stretched straight out in front of me. When I was in place, an IV needle was inserted into my left arm.

Now at the controls that would slowly draw me into the tube of death, the nice technician told me he was going to begin. He wasn't kidding that the MRI was loud. The only way one can hear what the technician says is through a speaker inside the machine. As I was drawn inside, I realized that God was filling that MRI with peace. Chaos seemed to reign outside, but inside, God provided me with the peace that surpasses understanding. It was comforting to hear Tim as he told me stories to keep my mind occupied. Between the earplugs and noise, I had no clue what he was saying, but I could hear his voice. I thought about how lambs know the voice of their shepherd. *The Lord is my Shepherd.* I praised God and thanked Him for helping me do this. I let go of the panic. I knew I needed to trust God.

"Half over," I heard.

What? No way, I thought. *I've only been in here a minute or two.*

As I lay there with my arms stretched out in front of me, I was reminded of the Man of Steel flying over Metropolis. I thought about a time when Rosa and I had gone to Madame Tussauds wax museum in New York. We made a video in which we were the superheroes flying over the city, protecting the citizens from unknown dangers. We were belly-down on a table with our arms outstretched, like I was now, in front of a green screen. Meteorites fell from the sky (NERF balls), and we had to use our superhuman strength to swat them away. We had so much fun that day; we laughed so hard that we were crying.

"All done!"

What? I wondered. *I've only been in here five minutes—seven, tops. Why did the technician lie to me about the length of the scan?*

Then I began to analyze that perhaps God had suspended time for me. Why not? He created time. He could do whatever He wanted. The technician took the IV out and slowly—slowly, as the bed inched out—I emerged from the cocoon of peace in which I had been enveloped. I thought about Shadrach, Meshach, and Abednego. These were three young Hebrew men who were taken captive by King Nebuchadnezzar. At that time, the king wanted all his subjects to worship a ninety-foot-tall statue of himself or be burned alive. These three knew there was only one choice. They had to be faithful to God and would not bow the knee to anyone but God.[5] They were probably scared to death. They were bound up[6] to be thrown into a fiery furnace, so hot that the flames killed the

---

[5] Daniel 3:1–18.
[6] Daniel 3: 21–22.

men who brought the trio up to the oven. Nevertheless, they trusted God in the face of great fear and peril and were protected from the inferno by God. Not only were they protected, but Jesus was right in the furnace with them.[7] Was He in the MRI with me? I pondered.

It was over! The events of the day left me very, very tired. I went home and took a hot bath—and *then* the Valium kicked in.

---

[7] Daniel 3:25.

Chapter 3

WHEN YOU KNOW GOD IS FOR YOU, IT DOESN'T MATTER WHO IS AGAINST YOU

I've heard that keeping a journal is helpful. I've often thought about it but never had the unction to do it. Yet during this journey I seemed drawn to write things down and have found it beneficial. At first, I used different colored pens and wrote in decorative fonts, but I've come to realize I don't have to get fancy. Simply writing down my thoughts and feelings got it out of my head and enabled me to remember everything God had done for me.

I drove to a local department store and purchased a handful of brightly colored notebooks. I included a Bible verse with each day's entry. On the front page of my first journal, I wrote, "who Himself bore our sins in His own body on the tree, that we, having died to sins, might live for righteousness—by whose stripes you were healed" (1 Peter 2:24). I taped a manila envelope to the back of the journal to store the cards I received. I labeled it "Blessings." Every prayer, every kind word, every thoughtful gesture meant the world to me. I wanted to remember each and every one.

My oldest daughter, Erin, is a BuJo (bullet journaling) journaler.

This type of daily logging allows you to organize everything from your thoughts to your daily schedule to your meal planning, using a bullet-style system. One might use charts and graphs, drawings, or just bullet points to highlight topics. Some of these journals can be very elaborate and quite beautiful, looking more like works of art than a journal. I tried doing that at first, but I had so many thoughts that it didn't work for me. I didn't always have the wherewithal to create a fanciful entry. Sometimes, I drew a picture to help illustrate what I meant. Other times, I might tape something to the page that I read that day, like a note from a friend or a page from the *Our Daily Bread* devotional. Whatever was in my noggin, I wanted out of me and on to paper. Once, I wrote about a dream I had. In it, my nose fell off, and I tried to stick it back on my face, but the process didn't look too promising. It sounded silly, but it made me laugh. I've come to realize that laughter is particularly good for your psyche, and if journaling about gluing my nose back on made me laugh, it was a good thing. "A merry heart does good, like medicine, But a broken spirit dries the bones" (Proverbs 17:22).

Once the results from the MRI were in, I had to go back to see Dr. Nett. He informed me that I had no lumps (yes, I'd heard that before), and the cancer hadn't spread to my lymph nodes (yay!); *however*, the masses were larger than originally thought. Therefore, he wanted to do the chemo first to shrink them. *Ugh!* I just wanted the cancer *out* of me.

Dr. Nett said the standard practice was to wait for surgery, as the chemo treatments can weaken, shrink, and even destroy breast cancer, so some woman may only need a lumpectomy instead of mastectomy.[8] That sounded logical. I prayed about all of this and thought it was a good plan of attack, and now it was just a matter of doing each thing, one step at a time. Nonetheless, I was a bit

---

[8] "Chemotherapy Before Surgery Increases Likelihood of Lumpectomy," Breastcancer.org, March 4, 2015, https://www.breastcancer.org/research-news/lumpectomy-after-neoadjuvant-chemo.

apprehensive about waiting for surgery, as I didn't want to pussyfoot around while this disease had a chance to fester and grow. I guess this weighed on me, as I was becoming an emotional wreck. Little things that went wrong somehow turned into big things. Insignificant experiences at work, which normally wouldn't have bothered me, brought me to tears. That's when I realized I wasn't OK. Simple things, like just trying to get the insurance forms filled out, became a huge to-do. For instance, I had to give the insurance provider my employee identification number. It's the same number I punch into the time clock every day, four times a day, five days a week, but for the life of me, I couldn't remember it. After I had pushed all the right prompts and waited so long to speak to a human being, I didn't want to hang up and start all over again, just because I was having a mental block. The woman on the other end of the phone was sweet and patient with me, but I was not patient with myself. I knew I was better than this and stronger than this. I was wrong.

One of the bumps in the road was a bit of static between Tim and me before the chemo treatments began. Tim felt helpless and wanted to *do* something to make me better, and he wasn't convinced traditional medicine was the answer. I wasn't happy about it, but I was comfortable with the treatment plan Dr. Nett had proposed to me. Through long discussions, much research, and listening to each other with loving ears, we came to a happy medium. I would go the traditional route, but we would integrate nutritional supplements and modify my eating habits to assist my immune system to fight this awful disease. We also asked many questions and voiced our concerns to my doctors. When I say *we*, I mean we talked it over and we prayed about it, but *I* ultimately had the final say. I know this was difficult for Tim, but he lovingly sat in the passenger's seat while I managed my treatment. For instance, Dr. Nett mentioned that one of my options was to have a contralateral prophylactic mastectomy. In other words, have my healthy breast removed as well as a preventive measure. Many women choose this option, as it greatly reduces the possibility of getting breast cancer again.

Actress Angelina Jolie had a double prophylactic mastectomy. She had not been diagnosed with cancer but had the procedure done as a preemptive strike, so to speak. Most cancer occurs by chance. Nevertheless, some people have a higher risk of developing cancer because of a gene mutation that runs in their families. Errors in two particular genes—BRCA1 and BRCA2—may increase a person's risk of certain types of cancer.[9] Angelina had a mutation in her BRCA1 gene. Having the double mastectomy proactively dropped her chance of getting cancer from 87 percent down to under 5 percent![10] I was ready to do this. Tim didn't want me to, but he never said a word. After much thought and prayer, however, I sensed God was directing me to keep my healthy breast. It was only after I announced my decision to Tim that he let out a huge sigh of relief and told me his true thoughts.

Concerned about my appointment with the oncologist the next day, I drew a self-portrait in my journal. I was visibly upset and stood beneath the sun, holding a rope lassoed to a rain cloud. Underneath the picture, I drew an old-fashioned fuse box that sparked, and I wrote the words "fuse overload." The picture was an illustration of what happens when we worry about tomorrow. I referenced Matthew 6:34—"Therefore do not worry about tomorrow, for tomorrow will worry about its own things. Sufficient for the day is its own trouble." Then I wrote, "When we worry about tomorrow, we pull tomorrow's clouds over today's sunshine." I was clinging to God's Word to give me hope and strength to face everything that was racing toward me at breakneck speed. I was afraid and felt alone and vulnerable.

Dr. Dawn's office was the antithesis of the radiology site. White walls, bright lights, no pictures on display, and a clock that was right only two times a day. The tiny examination room was no better. Tim

---

[9] Megan Hanson, MS, LGC, "What Are BRCA1 and BRCA2?," Healthpartners.com, https://www.healthpartners.com/blog/what-are-brca1-and-brca2.
[10] "Angelina Jolie and Other Celebs Focus Attention on BRCA Test," CBN.com, https://www1.cbn.com/healthyliving-17.

sat directly in front of me. There wasn't much to look at in the room, and the view of the parking lot from the third-floor window proved just as uninspiring. I imagined how a young, frightened woman might feel, sitting in this room. I had my supportive husband with me, but what about someone who was alone? What would be going through the mind of someone with young children? A mom could be sitting here, wondering if she'd be around to see her babies graduate high school. A married woman might be fearful that her husband wouldn't want her if she lost her hair and breasts. As I sat there on the exam table, with the crinkly white paper ripping underneath me, I saw something that bothered me. A pathetic, anemic-looking Christmas cactus, that was more dead than alive, was parked smack dab in the middle of the window sill. "What an awful thing to have in here!" I said, breaking the deafening silence and clearing the air of our thoughts. I wanted to help others, and I was going to start by making them throw out that decrepit plant.

As it turned out, Dr. Dawn was away, and her appointments were being covered by a noticeably young associate who was, no doubt, still wet behind the ears. She was all business and didn't smile. When she explained the treatment they were planning for me, it was very matter-of-fact. Ben Stein's voice in the movie *Ferris Bueller's Day Off* had more inflection. Her tone and demeanor were such that she could have been telling me the weather forecast. She gave me informational pamphlets, and I wouldn't have been surprised if the title of them was *The Proper Way to Have Cancer*. Everything was explained very clinically. I felt like she wasn't taking into consideration that I wasn't some test rat but a human being, with feelings and emotions. I'm certain that in med school, she was taught to have a posture of confidence in what she was saying and doing. To me, though, she emanated an air of superiority; *she* was the doctor, after all. I felt intimidated, and I didn't like it.

Both the surgeon and the oncologist explained to me that I would need to have a port surgically put in. This is a small piece of equipment that is implanted, usually on the right side of your chest, below the collar bone. It contains a tube that fits into a vein, as well as a port outside the vein, just under the skin, through which the oncologist injects the chemo. I was told that a port was preferable to infusing the chemo straight into a vein, as, on occasion, veins collapse. It also allows the drugs to be injected directly into your heart.[11] If you think this sounds extremely creepy, you're not alone. It's difficult to hear that this is what they want to do to you. I think, though, at this point, you kind of nod your head to whatever they tell you and try not to reflect on it too much.

She gave me several pamphlets to read, but those were just as frightening. I didn't want to add fuel to the already raging fire. I thought the information would just give me more anxiety because they tell you *anything and everything* that can go wrong. It's like those ads on television for various medications—while they're showing you a happy, beautiful woman and her adorable puppy running through a field of flowers, an announcer is quietly saying, "Some patients have reported losing limbs, unusual hair growth on their tongue, and barking like a rabid dog while taking this medicine. Side effects may include blindness, radical weight gain, and, on occasion, death."

I handed all the pamphlets to Tim and instructed him to read them. I just couldn't take it anymore. It was all too much to handle. I truly believed that God was going to deliver me from most of the ill effects. I even thought I might not lose my hair and that this journey would be a proverbial walk in the park.

The young oncologist said to advise the office when the port was being placed so an appointment could be made to have my first chemotherapy treatment that same day. Since all this was new to me, I didn't realize that although it was minor surgery, putting the

---

[11] "About Your Implanted Port," Memorial Sloan Kettering Cancer Center (MSKCC), last updated August 15, 2018, https://www.mskcc.org/cancer-care/patient-education/your-implanted-port.

port in was a big deal. In reality, there was no way I would be up to having chemo the same day I had surgery.

She also told me I needed to have tests done so the doctor could determine the course of treatment for me. That sounded good. I wanted a personal treatment plan, not something that was one-size-fits-all. The tests were an echocardiogram (EKG) to determine the health of my heart and a full-body scan to determine if I had cancer anywhere else. If I had been hooked up to the electrocardiograph monitor at that moment, they would have seen that my heart began racing at the mere mention of the word scan! I forced myself to remember how God had brought me through the MRI and tried not to panic.

After the exam, I was weighed and had blood drawn. There was a lab in the office, so they were able to analyze it and get back to me in a matter of minutes.[12] The nurse explained that the results were good (whatever that meant). I found out later that this was just to make sure I wasn't anemic and was healthy enough to receive the chemotherapy. Once I completed the EKG and body scan, Dr. Nett would insert the port. At that time, Dr. Dawn would decide which drug(s) she would use for my treatment. This was called a *protocol*, but I didn't know that either. There was a plethora of medical terminology for cancer with which I soon would become familiar, and it's a language I wished I didn't have to learn. Just for your reference, however, there is a dictionary of cancer terms that you might find helpful. It can be found at https://www.cancer.gov/publications/dictionaries/cancer-terms.

Along with the journaling, another tool I used as a coping mechanism was gathering prayer warriors to lift me up as I navigated these troubling waters. I felt vulnerable and needed women I knew I could trust who would intercede in prayer for me. I remembered the Bible book of Esther.

---

[12] "The Oncology Patient and Blood Counts," Genesis Convenient Care, https://www.genesishealth.com/care-treatment/cancer/resources/education/blood.

There's a long story about how Esther became queen, but there she was, married to the monarch of Persia (modern-day Iran), and she was in a predicament. An edict had been passed that decreed all the Jews would be annihilated, even the children. The king didn't know Esther was a Jew. She could have been spared any harm, had she just kept her mouth shut. But she couldn't do that. Esther knew she had to go to the king and plead for the lives of her people and, ultimately, hers as well. The twist here was that going into the king's presence without permission was a capital offense. Esther had not been called to stand before her husband for thirty days. If she went to see him, unsolicited, she knew it could mean her death. Esther was wise and didn't act without first preparing the way. She asked for help and requested her people fast for three days before she sought an audience with King Ahasuerus.[13] Although God is not mentioned in this book, it is implied that they sought His direct intervention through this fast. I too sought His intervention by contacting five or six female friends who I knew talked with God on a regular basis.

> Be anxious for nothing, but in everything by prayer and supplication, with thanksgiving, let your requests be made known to God. (Philippians 4:6)

These wonderful women not only lifted me up in prayer, but they sent encouraging scripture verses to motivate me. One woman immediately encouraged me to always remember that Christ, not cancer, was the "big C"! Over time, this lovely prayer circle widened to include so many people that I've lost count. Some would ask permission if they could share my prayer request with their Bible study group, or they'd inadvertently let it slip that I was ill, and then the people they told began praying for me. In addition, I asked the pastors (we have four) and elders of our church to anoint me with oil and pray over me, time and time again. James 5:14 says, "Is anyone

---

[13] Esther 4:16.

among you sick? Let him call for the elders of the church, and let them pray over him, anointing him with oil in the name of the Lord." Every Sunday, I made a practice of asking one of our ministers to pray over both Tim and me. If you are a churchgoer, you know how difficult it can be to speak to your pastor after service. Many a time, I had to wait, but I wouldn't leave without my blessing.

Right about now, you might think that cancer was my biggest battle. But God was also tearing down strongholds in my life. I'll explain what I mean. The word *strongholds* is found only once in the New Testament. It is a metaphor, used by the apostle Paul, to describe the spiritual battle of a Christian: "For though we walk in the flesh, we do not war according to the flesh. For the weapons of our warfare are not carnal but mighty in God for pulling down strongholds" (2 Corinthians 10:3–4). To be truly free, God graciously removes things that have kept us prisoners, whether it's fear, hate, pain, or whatever. Claustrophobia has been an albatross around my neck as far back as I can remember. I kept it a secret for decades, until I realized it was irrational, and I had no control over it. I reasoned I was a helpless victim. I've been asked on many occasions if I ever was stuck in an elevator. No. And never have I been locked in a closet or detained against my will—that is, until May fourth.

The day started out great. It was *Star Wars* day (May the fourth be with you). I was at work, and I needed to get supplies from what my coworkers referred to as *the vault*. It was a windowless interior room that was locked and alarmed and had limited access. Along with money, certain expensive supplies were kept there. The door to enter the vault led to a dark, windowless hallway. (They have since installed lights.) The walls were made of cold, hard cinder blocks. The door at the other end was locked, and although the door I came through was not, I still felt closed in when I shut it.

I was pacing in front of the outer door when a coworker approached me and asked if I had a problem. I explained that I was severely claustrophobic and going into the vault hallway was stressful. He told me that his father had the same malady; the only way to get over it, he said, was to face it. He then approached me so closely that he stood on my toes. I remember this distinctly because my feet were sore, and my toes throbbed under his weight. He put his face as close to mine as he could without touching me and said, "How do you feel now? Do you feel closed in now?"

I stepped back and put both of my hands up and out to indicate *stop*! I wanted my body language to reflect what I was saying. "No! I'm fine. I'm out in the open."

His facial expression changed, and I erroneously took that to mean he was sorry. He offered to go in with me, but I told him no.

"Please don't," I said, again raising my hands in front of me.

He was insistent; he put his arm around me and guided me into the hallway. I thought he was trying to make up for his inappropriate behavior and help me. Regrettably, what he did next was heartless! Once inside the hallway, he shut the door very forcefully and stood in front of it with his hands behind him, still on the doorknob. "What are you going to do?" he said with a grin. "Are the walls caving in on you now?"

I tried to push him to get to the doorknob, but he wouldn't budge. It was hard to see in the dark hallway, but I could tell he enjoyed what he was doing as he was grinning. He pushed me away from the door, which prompted me to start screaming. After what seemed like an eternity, I was able to push him out of the way. I was still screaming when I came out of the hallway. I was shaking and crying and didn't know what to do. To make a long story short, he got to Human Resources before I did and lied about the whole incident. Since there were no eyewitnesses, it was my word against his. The malicious actions he put on display that day shook me to the core. I was already feeling vulnerable and helpless, and this only added to my self-loathing. Why did I let fear dictate my actions?

At day's end, even though I was not in the proper frame of mind, I headed to the hospital for my tests. The CT was done in an open-air scanner, which was a blessing. I took a much-needed nap when we got home. While I was sleeping, Tim called everyone to keep them up-to-date, and again, he had a tiff with Rupert. (*Sigh*.) I had my own fears and distress to deal with, and I just couldn't be the referee every time someone else got upset because of my condition. Whether it was my physical ailments or mental upheaval, I was treading in uncharted territory and had a difficult time just dealing with *me*. I was unprepared to handle anyone else's problems. I fervently tried to avoid drama; nevertheless, it managed to find me. I was emotionally frazzled.

Simple things that I thought would be a no-brainer somehow managed to turn into nightmares. One such incident was a visit to a doctor. The same-day surgery to have my port implanted was scheduled. The only thing standing between me and this surgery was the *special dispensation* I needed from my general practitioner, saying I was physically fit. This type of appointment typically took no more than half an hour. The last time I'd visited this office, I was treated by a fast-acting, no-nonsense dedicated physician, which was in contrast to the doctor I found myself impatiently waiting (and waiting) for during this appointment. As requested, I arrived fifteen minutes early, only to sit forty-five additional minutes before being called in to the examination room. I was left in a tiny airless room, in a paper gown, alone with my thoughts for thirty more minutes. It was early May, but the weather felt more like summer than spring. I'd had enough! I was sweaty, tired, hungry, and frustrated. I walked to the receptionists' desk, holding the opening of the flimsy gown shut so my bits and pieces didn't hang out, and asked them when the doctor was going to grace me with his presence. If there was a problem and he was detained, a little forewarning would have been nice. I felt forgotten and unimportant. The receptionist apologized profusely and tried to explain that this doctor always ran late. She guided me back to the exam room and opened the window. This was helpful, as I was there for another fifteen before he finally showed up. By then, I was a wreck; my hands were shaking, and I was not happy. You must remember that my alarm was set for 3:45 each morning, so by 7:00 p.m., I am fried. Well, Dr. Tardypants, as I choose to call him, sauntered in and was as cool as a cucumber. We began the usual doctor-patient discussion, and he noticed that I was upset. "How much do you drink?" he asked nonchalantly.

"Listen," I said firmly. "A month ago, I was fine. Since then, I've found out I have cancer, and it's been a whirlwind of medical appointments and tests. Yes, I'm upset. Wouldn't anyone be?"

Again, Dr. Tardypants, without looking up from the computer screen, explained that I could benefit from antidepressants. Many cancer patients used them, he explained matter-of-factly. I thought my head was going to explode! After that incident, I made sure I never saw Dr. Tardypants again. One of the biggest criteria I have for medical professionals is that they are caring. I think that if they have honest concern for their patients, they will automatically provide patients with the best treatment they possible can. It is very frustrating to put your trust in a person who has sworn to "do no harm," yet treats you like a second-class citizen. In my case, I felt it would be better if I considered it a learning experience and let it go. I didn't want to waste my energy on nonsense. In the end, he wasn't part of my cancer treatment team, so no harm, no foul.

Chapter 4

KNOWING THE BIBLE IS ONE THING; KNOWING THE AUTHOR IS ANOTHER

I now knew what a ping-pong ball felt like, as I bounced back and forth from one doctor to another. This time, I was visiting the oncologist to get the rundown of what was to come. I went to the appointment, armed with a healthy baby spider plant. It was a cutting from a larger plant I humorously had named Power. When we checked in, I presented the receptionist with Power Jr., which was planted in a bright lime-green ceramic pot, complete with care instructions. I strongly advised her to deposit the dead thing in the exam room into the nearest trash receptacle.

Our wait wasn't long before we finally got to meet Dr. Dawn. I was apprehensive at first because of the experience with her associate and what Dr. Nett had said about her. But I soon realized she was very approachable and didn't mind answering any and all questions. She was about five foot two, always wore a smile, and was soft-spoken with a slight British accent. I also found her to be very grandmotherly.

I told her I was scheduled to have my port put in and gave her the date so she could pencil me in for an appointment on the same day (as instructed by her associate). Dr. Dawn chuckled and told us she would see us the week after, as I had to wait until I was healed. The newbie oncologist, who was shadowing the doctor, interjected how important it was to receive the chemo, as it was "very expensive." (This was another clue to me that she was still wet behind the ears when it came to her doctor/patient skills.) Very calmly, Dr. Dawn gestured with her hand to the junior physician, as if to silence her, and assured us that she had my best interest at heart, and I shouldn't worry about dates and times. She wanted me to be well first before the treatments began.

I was asked if I wanted to take the genetic test to see if I carried the BRCA gene. To do this, I had to provide a saliva sample. A mutated BRCA gene could be passed down to my children, and that worried me. I didn't let on to any of my girls that I had done this until I got the results. I figured there was no need to worry them unnecessarily.

To take this test, you are asked to swish a rinse around in your mouth that works to collect cells. In my case, it was a tiny bottle of mouthwash. I then had to spit it back into a container that was sent off to a lab for analysis. It was bad enough getting cancer. I couldn't bear the heartache if my children had inherited anything from me that might increase their chances of getting this awful disease.

Dr. Dawn told me I would lose my hair in about a month and gave me a prescription for a wig, or hair prosthesis, as it is medically called. I still didn't believe I would go bald, but I took the 'script anyway.

With all that behind me, it was off to see Dr. Nett ... again. He wanted to explain the procedure for implanting the port. I wanted to learn all about it. Surgery didn't scare me. What concerned me the most about operations was being anesthetized. I detest being nauseated, but then, who doesn't? Dr. Nett calmed my fears when he told me it would be twilight anesthesia. He explained that I wouldn't be totally *under*, but I wouldn't care or feel pain. Technically, twilight sleep is a mild dose of sedation that relieves anxiety and gives you anterograde amnesia (the inability to form new memories). Since I wouldn't be unconscious, he clarified, I should not feel nauseated.

I wanted to know everything about this port. I asked many questions, but I still came home and looked it up on the internet. I wanted to know what it would look like once it was in me. I was sure I'd see a few horror stories, but I thought I knew enough to sort out fact from fiction. Yikes! What I learned was that things sometimes go wrong. Many of the pictures I saw were terrifying. So for this specific procedure, I decided to limit my investigating to the American Cancer Society's website. I just wanted the facts about what was going to happen, not every narrative that ended in a malpractice suit.

The day of my operation arrived, and, true to Dr. Nett's word, I emerged from the surgical suite feeling great. No nausea. Yay! I had a large bandage over the site where the port now resided. The nurses kept telling me that when the numbing medicine wore off, I would be very sore. So, anticipating pain, I took a Percocet when I got home. Bad idea! Number one, I really wasn't hurting that bad so I probably would have been fine taking acetaminophen; and number two, all the Percocet did was make me sick. That defeated the whole purpose of the twilight sleep. Note to self: *never* take Percocet again!

Two days later I was able to return to work. Once again, I didn't sleep well. My mind was preoccupied with worry about the upcoming chemo treatment, suffering from *funds-a-low* and losing my job. Even though it's not a fabulous career, I didn't want to get fired for being out so often. We needed the money, and, more importantly, I needed the health insurance. Ultimately, I know God provides, and He would have arranged for something else, had my employment been terminated. Tim saw my distress and sat by my bedside and spoke calmly to me as he stroked my back. That made all the difference and calmed my nerves so I was able to sleep. It's comforting to know you are loved.

The next morning, as I dragged my tired, wretched body to

work, I tried not to feel sorry for myself. However, there was a raging pity party going on inside of my head—that is, until God introduced me to someone. If you haven't surmised by now, I worked in retail. Early in the day, a woman approached me and asked for help finding a particular item. One look at her and my whole perspective changed. This sweet woman was a burn victim. Her face was terribly scarred. She had no eyelashes, eyebrows, or lips. I could see that it was difficult for her move her mouth to speak. Nevertheless, there she was, standing in front of me, with all the courage in the world to go out in public and not be ashamed to approach a stranger. She held her head high. I didn't know this woman, but I immediately felt such admiration for her. I looked her in the eyes, smiled, and offered her the best help I could. My cancer could be cut out. Her scars were forever. Shame on me!

Later that same day, I heard about a terrible traffic accident on a nearby highway involving a school bus, resulting in the death of a fifth-grade child. I thought about the parents of that child and how they would do anything, including getting cancer, just to hold their baby, safe and sound, in their arms again. I prayed for these parents, and I asked God to please forgive me and give me an attitude of gratitude. That night, I wrote this verse in my journal: "Whoever offers praise glorifies Me" (Psalm 50:23a).

I also tried to concentrate on the *whatevers* that are in Philippians 4:8:

> Finally, brethren, whatever things are true, whatever things are noble, whatever things are just, whatever things are pure, whatever things are lovely, whatever things are of good report, if there is any virtue and if there is anything praiseworthy—meditate on these things.

It's easy to be drawn down into a pit of despair when you concentrate only on the negatives. Yes, I needed to think positively, but don't take that to mean that I subscribed to the *religion* of positive thinking. What I mean by that is, there are people who try to use their own power or that of a nebulous higher power (the universe, for example) to achieve what they want. This religion is based on the individual's actions. Its philosophy—that individuals are solely responsible for their feelings—doesn't leave room for human weaknesses. Neither does it take into consideration the spiritual realm. There are evil forces at work that would like nothing more than to see us fail. Faith, on the other hand, relies on God's power and what *He* wants. Faith isn't about us; it's realizing that our strength comes from the one true God. Positive thinking alone is all about the creation and satisfying us; what *we think* is good. In contrast, faith glorifies God and wants His will for our lives. What He has in mind is worlds different than what we think. "'For My thoughts are not your thoughts, Nor are your ways My ways,' says the Lord" (Isaiah 55:8).

I don't share that to put anyone down but to shout the good news! It's not up to us. We don't have to shoulder the burden to make sure things work out. Jesus bore it all when He died on the cross in our place. If we mess up (and as human beings, that's a guarantee), we can know that we have a definite, real, true *someone* who is in control and who loves us! How wonderful! I can rely on the sovereign Author of life to work everything out *for my good*.[14] That said, thinking positive thoughts was not enough for me. I needed power in my life. I knew I couldn't do this on my own. I was not convinced that visualizing a positive outcome was enough. Again, turning to God's Word for encouragement and strength, I read, "And do not be conformed to this world, but be transformed by the renewing of your mind, that you may prove what is that good and acceptable and perfect will of God" (Romans 12:2).

God wanted to be more than a *concept* of a divine being to me.

---

[14] "And we know that all things work together for good to those who love God, to those who are the called according to His purpose" (Romans 8:28).

He wanted me to genuinely know Him and live in His *realness*. He's not a lucky rabbit's foot to rub when you're in trouble or want something. He wants us to have a *true* relationship with Him because He cares for us.

I thought about my girls and my Tim, and I thanked God for all the wonderful cheerleaders He placed in my life who cared for me, were praying for me, and were rooting for me. Yes, I was afraid—very afraid—but not that I would die; I was afraid of the ordeal I had to go through. This was not at all what I had planned. Still, I had peace, knowing God was directing everything, and I was in the palm of His hand. That is what made all the difference.

I am reminded of Corrie ten Boom, author of the book *The Hiding Place*. The first fifty years of her life were uneventful. She was a single woman who made watches in her father's shop in Holland. However, when the Nazis invaded and occupied the Netherlands, her life was forever changed. God chose to use a middle-aged, unassuming Corrie and her family to save hundreds of people from certain death. The ten Booms secretly built a hidden room in their tiny house to conceal Jewish refugees as they fled from the bloodthirsty regime. When it was discovered that they were helping Jews escape, the family was arrested and sent to a concentration camp. There, all but Corrie died. Yet, she said, "Jesus did not promise to change the circumstances around us. He promised great peace and pure joy to those who would learn to believe that God actually controls all things."

I was learning that.

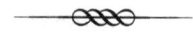

With prescriptions in hand, I went to the drugstore to get what I needed for my first infusion of chemo. The pharmacist informed me that the antinausea medication alone was going to cost me five hundred dollars! We immediately called the doctor and explained the problem to her. We didn't know how to proceed. The office encouraged us to keep the appointment. So, on a beautiful, sunny spring morning, we headed off to see Dr. Dawn. After being weighed and having my blood drawn and analyzed, I was ready to begin. The nurse who attended to me was sweet and friendly. She tried to make this experience pleasant and wanted me to look at it as a positive event. To this day, I still can't picture chemotherapy in a positive light. It was a horrible feeling, being hooked up to an IV that held the bright red toxin. Ironically, the drug is called Adriamycin.

We were there for a few hours. The machine that doled out the chemo made a rhythmic humming sound. The only distraction from it was a small television mounted to the wall, but it was daytime TV, and I didn't want to watch *Divorce Court* or soap operas. I brought pictures of my grandsons to cheer me up. Blaise's contagious smile beamed out at me from his kindergarten class picture, and River was still cooking in his mommy's belly so his was a grainy ultrasound image. I'd also packed my journal in my bag of goodies, but it was too difficult to write. My hands were shaking, and I was distracted. The only thing I managed to get down on paper was, "The angel of the Lord encamps all around those who fear Him, And delivers them" (Psalm 34:7).

Most of the patients I met there were happy to get the treatments because, to them, it meant they were going to get better. It was hope. Some of the poor people I met had death written all over them. Their skin was gray, they had no hair, and they walked slowly, bent over, determined to get their next treatment. I, however, felt like I was voluntarily swallowing poison. Adriamycin is so powerful that there are warnings issued to keep your body fluids from coming in contact with others.[15] You are instructed to wash any soiled clothing immediately and to use gloves when touching *your own* body's fluids for at least five days after each treatment. I received other medicines as well, but that's the one I remember—or should I say, I'll never

---

[15] "Adriamycin," Drugs.com, last updated September 27, 2020, https://www.drugs.com/cdi/adriamycin.html.

forget. I found out later that medical personnel have given this particular chemo drug the nickname "Red Devil."

While I sat tethered to the infusion pump, I was told to drink plenty of water. That also meant plenty of trips to the little girls' room. Tim sat with me for those long hours, talking to me, getting water bottles, and helping me navigate back and forth to the bathroom. He made sure the wires from the pump didn't get tangled up or caught on anything and became a real pro at it. One of the medications I received intravenously was Benadryl. This helped to alleviate any allergic reaction to the chemotherapy medications, and it made me drowsy. I was afraid I was going to miss more days from work than I wanted to. *As long as I don't get nauseated, I'm good*, I thought.

One of the first medicines I got intravenously was to prevent nausea; therefore, I felt great while I was at the doctor's office. When we got home, however, I began to feel queasy, and the next thing I knew, I was vomiting. This continued for about a week. I didn't realize that much time had passed and couldn't understand why Tim was so worried. Of course, I had nothing left in me to throw up, but the dry heaves continued. About three days into this ordeal, Tim brought me back to the oncologist's office to be rehydrated. So here was the *ray of sunshine*, going into the office, hunched over a small wastebasket (in case I *whoopsed*, as my mother used to call it). I was angry that they let me go ahead with the treatment without the antinausea medication. I was frustrated that I couldn't even help myself; how was I going to help anyone else?

The sweet nurse who had given me the chemo wasn't in that day, but I met another nurse; I'll call her Nurse X. She told me that no matter how I felt, I shouldn't give in to the urge to vomit, as it was all in my head. She informed me that the rest of the treatments were going to be bad, but it was the only way I was going to get better, and I should fight it. Boy, that sure wasn't what I wanted to hear. I wanted comforting words and something to ease the pain in my gut. When I came home, I was still miserable, still had dry heaves, and still didn't want to eat or drink anything.

Finally, a week after my treatment, I began to see the light at the end of the tunnel. I was able to eat some soup and drink some bland tea. However, because I had been out from work for more than five days, I was automatically put on disability leave. I also found out that my insurance company did, in fact, cover the antinausea meds, but we were in a pharmacy that wasn't in the network. Had we gone across the street to another drugstore, we would have gotten everything I needed right away and at an affordable price.

A funny thing about those seven days of being so very sick was that I had amazing peace. After five days of heaving, I was finally able to write in my journal. I wrote down the lyrics from a hymn—"Then sings my soul, my Savior God, to Thee, how great Thou art!"[16]—along with a verse from 2 Corinthians 4:16: "Therefore we do not lose heart. Even though our outward man is perishing, yet the inward man is being renewed day by day."

I made a note that if I died, I wanted a choir, *in robes*, with tambourines, singing at my funeral service. (I have a running joke with our music director at church that we need choir robes for our singers. He just rolls his eyes and smiles.)

I started feeling better but was frustrated at how sick I had been. When I was well enough, I wrote in my journal, with tears streaming down my cheeks:

> The Hope of the Faithful, and the Messiah's Victory
> A Michtam of David.
> Preserve me, O God, for in You I put my trust.
> (Psalm 16:1)
>
> The Lord will fight for you, and you shall hold your peace. (Exodus 14:14)

---

[16] "How Great Thou Art" was based on a poem written by Swedish poet and pastor Carl Bober in 1885, titled "O Store Gud," or "O Mighty God."

Then, I decided to write my own psalm:

A Psalm of Hope

Lord, help me as I cry out. Things besiege me that I cannot control. Invisible enemies seek me out to kill my spirit. The pain enters my bones and I cry aloud.

Too weak to rise from my bed. Too ill to take nourishment, and yet there is a loud song that only I can hear streaming from my heart loud, strong, powerful, steadfast *shalom*!

I was weak, helpless, angry, hurt, and sore, but I was blessed. I had such peace and gratitude and was humbled by the experience. Physically, it was absolutely awful, but my spirit was rejoicing. I could truly say, "God is good."

So many times, I have heard people say that after hearing of a happy or positive event. "I just got a raise! God is good!" Yes, that is true, but God is good even when I am absolutely miserable, and things don't seem to be going well. God's goodness does not change with my circumstances.

Chapter 5

JESUS LOVES ME, LOVES ME STILL; THOUGH I'M WEAK AND VERY ILL

I absolutely adore warm weather, and it was beautiful outside. The birds were singing, the sun was shining, and flowers were blooming in our yard. If I had to be sick, I was glad I could convalesce in the spring and summer. We live in an area that is very natural and rustic. Our home is on what's called a "paper road." It's indicated on paper, but in reality, it's usually just a footpath. We don't even have a street sign signifying that there sorta kinda is a road here. There's a wooded yard, where many animals wander in and out. We've seen bear on occasion but mostly deer, raccoons, wild turkeys, foxes, a stray cat or two, and a wide variety of birds, including a pileated woodpecker. My favorite room in the house is our Florida room, or, as we call it, the Garden of Eatin'. There are windows on three sides of the room, giving us a terrific panoramic view of the lake, sixty feet or so below us. The room is chock-full of plants, including Audrey (named after the ginormous alien plant in *Little Shop of Horrors*) that we think is a fan palm. When I got her, she was barely two and a half feet high. In four years' time, however, she grew to about eight feet tall. In one corner, we have an antique *truhe* (pronounced *true*-uh, the German word for chest) that Tim acquired in Germany when he was in the army during the Vietnam War. I made a cushion for it and covered some extra-large pillows to make an inviting corner to sit with a book or just gaze out the windows at the lake and its goings-on. It's small but serene. Swans, ducks, cranes, and—once in a blue moon—an otter can be seen enjoying themselves on the water. The section of the lake near us is a no-wake zone, so the only boats we see are slow-moving pontoon boats, rowboats, canoes, kayaks and sailboats.

Our dining area is in this delightful room. We have a Narnia table and chairs. We call it this because it is fanciful. It's made of iron, although it looks more like pewter, and is ornate. It has a glass top and scroll-like legs with open swirling designs that are reminiscent of C. S. Lewis's imaginary world on the other side of the wardrobe. We found this set at Curb-Mart and decided to cover the chairs with bright tropical-colored paisley fabric. The pillows on the truhe match the cushions, and the plant pots throughout the room echo these colors. I also used the turquois, orange, red, and lime green to accent a second-hand table that I painted, which sits on the far side of the room. We snaked artificial ivy entwined with small white Christmas tree lights around the tops of the windows. When the sun goes down and the lights come on, you get the feeling of being in an open-air café. Over the years, we've picked up lanterns that hang from the ceiling here and there, adding to the room's quaintness. Two of the lanterns we bought while in the Caribbean and were made by local craftsmen. They share the bright warm colors of our little oasis on the hill and are shaped to look like tropical fish. Our fishy napkin holders are also preowned, and I painted them to have splashes of these whimsical colors.

I tease Tim by telling him I was switched at birth and was supposed to be a tropical princess. "You see," I tell him, "there was a Jamaican woman having a baby at the same time as my mother, and I was given to the wrong mom. Meanwhile, the Jamaican woman went back to her beautiful tropical paradise with her new baby in tow, and I'm stuck in the Garden State."

He is amazed that after living in the temperate climate of New Jersey all my life, I still have not acclimated to it. I have not, and when I was undergoing chemotherapy treatment, it got worse. I found that my thermometer was broken so I could not regulate my body's temperature. When I was warm, I would drink a frosty-cold smoothie made with yogurt, fruit, milk, and lots of ice. If I was cold, I had to take a warm bath or venture outside to sit in the sun. This room became a welcome escape for me. We decided it was a cancer-free room, and all talk of doctors, sickness, and the like would not be mentioned in this part of the house.

I was so discouraged by the fiasco of the last treatment that I began to have disturbing nightmares—that is, when I was able to sleep. I would wake up in the middle of the night, shaking, because I was so terrified. I have never been so afraid in my life. In my dreams, I would be strapped to a chair in Dr. Dawn's office, where I was being given a chemo cocktail against my will. It was like a torture chamber. I'd wake up in a start, get out of bed, and turn on gospel music to calm myself. It also helped to read from my devotional. One night, my reading suggested I look to the horizon (something sailors say to help those getting seasick to gain a sense of perspective), but I wasn't sure how to do that. I felt defeated and knew I just couldn't *do* this. So much for being strong.

Side effects from the chemo began to crop up, like pain in my mouth. I got nervous that I'd start losing my teeth. I also noticed that I couldn't think straight. It was sometimes hard to string a sentence together. Simple words eluded me. Once, I was trying to tell Tim about weighing myself, and I couldn't, for the life of me, remember the simple, everyday word *scale*. I remembered my mother participated in something called aerobics of the mind. The group at her senior center would tackle word games and number puzzles to keep their cognitive abilities sharp. I decided I would do that too. I found out later that this mental fuzziness is dubbed *chemo brain* (not a medical term). It's not unusual for patients undergoing chemotherapy treatment to suffer some sort of cognitive impairment or dysfunction. I needed help. I wrote Hebrews 4:16 in my journal that day: "Let us therefore come boldly to the throne of grace, that we may obtain mercy and find grace to help in time of need."

So although things weren't going as planned or smoothly, I could *know* I'd be OK. I had confidence that anything that happened to me was by design and for my good. This awareness was invaluable. The chorus from a hymn written by Bill Gaither, titled "Because He Lives," resonates this sentiment exactly:

> Because He lives, I can face tomorrow,
> Because He lives, all fear is gone
> Because I know He holds the future
> And life is worth the living, just because He lives

The results of the BRCA test were negative! I called my girls to give them the good news. As I said earlier, I hadn't told them I took the test because I didn't want to worry them needlessly. I felt such a sense of relief when Dr. Dawn gave me the report. I was happy to be able to say something positive to my children.

Regrettably, the knowledge that I had three more months of chemo hung over me like the sword of Damocles. It was just ten days after my introduction to chemo, and I was supposed to go back to the oncologist for my second dose. I was so petrified that I shook. I took the time before the appointment to pray while walking in the yard, repeating Psalm 34:7 over and over. I asked God to deliver me from this dreadful poison. I was getting physically sick just thinking about being hooked up to the IV.

When we got to the doctor's office, I asked Tim to please let me do the speaking. I wanted Dr. Dawn to know just how upset *I* was that I had been given the chemo without antinausea meds. I was angry that Nurse X had insinuated my pain and vomiting were all in my head. I ranted on to both the nurse (not Nurse X, as she wasn't there) and doctor, who patiently listened to everything I had to say. They didn't interrupt me, and they understood why I was so troubled. They both apologized profusely, and Dr. Dawn discussed altering my protocol so I would have fewer side effects. She gently suggested I try the Adriamycin one more time (*with* the antinausea meds). She also said she'd give me another week to relax and feel better. She could see I was agitated and anxious and wanted me to calm down.

As you can plainly see, my journey was not a smooth ride. Unfortunately, I doubt very highly that anyone's journey through this is smooth. Therefore, I wanted to do something pleasant after this debacle and decided to get my hair prosthesis before I needed it. I located a business that specialized in providing wigs for those affected by medical-related hair loss. Because they catered to sick women, it was by appointment only. This way, each customer had their undivided attention, and they personally could attend to her specific needs.

The center was about an hour's drive, as the crow flies, and I was tense before we even started the trip. The whole idea of losing my hair was humiliating and embarrassing, but if I was going to go bald, I wanted to have a wig available. There was no way I was going to walk around with a turban on my head. Some women look elegant or exotic with a scarf or head covering, but I am *not* one of those women.

Tim's opinion of my getting a wig was quite the opposite. He did not want to go to the center. When we prepare to head out somewhere, Tim is typically late. This isn't done purposefully; he is just time-challenged. The hands on the clock somehow move faster when he's trying to get out the door. On that day, however, he made no bones about his intentions. He resisted getting out of bed when the alarm went off and hit the snooze button like he was playing whack-a-mole. He was frustrated and agitated. The littlest thing on the drive there—like a wrong turn or a red light—put him into a tailspin. He uncharacteristically got short with me. Tim saw what the chemo did after just one dose and didn't want to think about what might happen next time. He didn't want there to be a next time and saw my wig as my acceptance of my treatment. When we finally arrived, not only were we half an hour late, but I was carsick. *Just perfect.*

The center was a cozy little house that had been converted into a haven for sick women. The homey features and atmosphere were calming and made my visit less strained. The decor was soft and feminine, kind of a romantic Victorian feel. The ladies who worked there were caring and sweet. Even though we missed half of our appointment, they didn't rush us. When my tummy calmed down, we all went upstairs to a room that was lined with shelves that held wig after wig after wig. When I saw all the mannequin heads, I gasped and felt like crying. It was overwhelming to see all the emotionless faces staring at me, like some strange *Twilight Zone* episode. I tried to make a joke to cut the tension, but it didn't work.

None of the wigs was me. They were all perfect. My hair, since I was a baby, was anything but perfect. It was thick and wavy and had a mind of its own. If I put on any of these wigs, I'd look like I was wearing a wig. I sat down in the seat of honor before a large mirror. The nice lady explained about the wigs, the price ranges, and how they could be ordered in different colors. She helped me try on a few, and I was embarrassed because my hair was brittle and really looked a mess. Unbeknownst to me, I was already starting to lose my hair. It had been falling out so much that, later, Tim told me it had clogged up the vacuum. I guess I would have had the Yul Brenner look much sooner, but because my hair was so thick, it took longer to fall out. Tim and I both agreed that these wigs weren't right. I didn't think I'd find anything that I would be comfortable wearing.

Then I looked up and saw it. It was the only hairpiece sitting on a small shelf right above the mirror. It was also the only wig that looked like it had survived a tornado. "That's it!" I said as I pointed to it. The nice lady smiled as she put the wig on my head. We all knew right away that this was the one. When I looked at my reflection, I saw *me*.

This wig was synthetic, so unlike a human-hair wig, there was no need to worry about curling or straightening it. The wig looked how it looked, and that was that. Even after washing it, the *hair* would revert to this shape all by itself. I was, however, warned against wearing my wig while cooking because the heat could damage it. That's one of the main differences between the two types of wigs. Also, the price tag on human-hair wigs started at $1,000. If a woman suffers from alopecia (a condition that currently has no cure, in which the immune system attacks hair follicles and causes hair loss), she might choose to invest in a more natural-feeling human-hair wig. Insurance covered a good portion of the cost of my new 'do, and I was grateful for that.

Tim apologized for his behavior and how it had stressed me out, but I understood. We were both emotionally beat up and didn't want to admit to ourselves that it was going to get worse before it got better.

In our *infinite wisdom*, we also made a dentist appointment for that day. One stressful event wasn't enough. I was concerned about my teeth, as I was experiencing pain whenever I ate. After x-rays and a thorough exam, the dentist proclaimed that my teeth and gums were fine. The pain was a reaction from the chemo. He suggested I eat alkaline food and "drink, drink, drink water!" He also told me something I wouldn't have expected from a dentist—"Suck on hard candy." He explained that this would trigger my glands to release more saliva, and that was good for my teeth and gums.

The days were long, now that I wasn't working every day. I did a lot of reading and writing and remembered putting Exodus 14:14 in my journal after my chemo treatment: "The Lord will fight for you, and you shall hold your peace." I wanted to find out the context of this verse, so I read the biblical account of the exodus of the children of Abraham from Egypt. I'm sure you are familiar with the story. I'm almost positive that most people have seen Cecil B. DeMille's epic 1956 film, *The Ten Commandments*. But here's a quick rundown: the Hebrews were slaves in Egypt for four hundred years and cried out to God for deliverance. God heard them and inflicted ten plagues upon Egypt (to show the Hebrews His divine power). After that, Pharaoh told Moses and Aaron to "Get out!"[17] Where would they go? They had no highways, road signs, or GPS to direct them. However, God didn't just free them and leave them. He was their guide. Wherever God guides, He provides.

> And the Lord went before them by day in a pillar of cloud to lead the way, and by night in a pillar of fire to give them light, so as to go by day and night. He did not take away the pillar of cloud by day or the pillar of fire by night from before the people. (Exodus 13:21–22)

Pretty amazing, right? They could travel by day and night. Remember, there were no streetlights back then. When the sun went down, *it got dark*. But wait—Pharaoh was not done with the Hebrews just yet, and he (and his army) chased after them.[18] Not such a fair fight. These were seasoned soldiers, with horses and chariots, prepared for battle. This had the Hebrews quaking in their sandals.[19]

Now the children of Abraham were in a real predicament. They were hemmed in, with mountains on one side and the Red Sea on another, and right behind them was a horde of Egyptians, bound

---

[17] Exodus 12:31.
[18] Exodus 14:9.
[19] Exodus 14:10.

and determined to slaughter them all. They were in a very scary place, but it was exactly where God wanted them to be, and He protected them. (I needed to remember that every time I was in a scary place.) But instead of trusting God, who had just performed some amazing wonders right in front of their very eyes, they turned on the man who was trying to save them.

> Then they said to Moses, "Because there were no graves in Egypt, have you taken us away to die in the wilderness? Why have you so dealt with us, to bring us up out of Egypt? Is this not the word that we told you in Egypt, saying, 'Let us alone that we may serve the Egyptians'? For it would have been better for us to serve the Egyptians than that we should die in the wilderness." (Exodus 14:11–12)

I thought, *Wait a minute! What are they talking about? The Hebrews begged God to free them!* Then I noticed something as I read this passage; by looking at the Egyptians, they had to look right past God (remember the pillar of cloud and pillar of fire? It had moved between the newly-freed Hebrews and the Egyptians). No wonder they were afraid. They weren't looking at their source of strength and remembering all the miracles He did to liberate them. They instead were focusing on the situation around them. How many times had I done that? Instead of remembering what God already had done for me and looking to my Deliverer, I looked at my situation.

Now we get to the whole reason I looked this up:

> And Moses said to the people, "Do not be afraid. Stand still, and see the salvation of the Lord, which He will accomplish for you today. For the Egyptians whom you see today, you shall see again no more forever. The Lord will fight for you, and you shall hold your peace." (Exodus 14:13–14)

God was, yet again, going to perform a miraculous act to save His people. They didn't have to lift a finger—no battle, no casualties of war, no work on their part to defeat the enemy. God took care of it all. Great, right? Well, I guess I'm not too far removed from the Hebrews because it's not always so easy for me to do either. How many times had I looked around at my circumstances and thought things were hopeless? I wrote this prayer in my journal:

> Lord, may I look at Your Glory when I face hard, scary times. May I "remember" your mighty deeds of the past and trust in You.

Chapter 6

I KNOW SO

Hair—we take it for granted. At least, I did. I always had thick, unruly hair. When I was little, my mother didn't know what to do with it. The best she could do was a ponytail or pigtails. I always admired the African American girls in school who had stunning hairstyles, beautiful waves, curls, and elaborate braids. My hair was always wild and all over my head.

Now, I was faced with losing my hair, and I wasn't sure how I felt about it. I take that back. I felt unattractive. Add to that the lack of eyebrows and eyelashes, and I really felt ugly. I found myself admiring other women who had shiny, healthy hair. They didn't know how blessed they were. Every day, my hair got thinner and thinner. It felt and looked like it had been burned. It was brittle and frizzy, which, in turn, made my scalp itch. Part of me wanted to lose the hair, just so I'd be comfortable, but the other part of me wanted my long, healthy hair back. As I washed my hair, it didn't seem to be connected to my head very well. I thought it would fall out in dribs and drabs. Boy, was I wrong.

Even though I was going through a tough time, I realized that

Tim was going through his own pain. Everyone put their focus on me, but I was worried about him. He had to pick up all the pieces, and he did it so I wouldn't worry. For instance, he kept the ever-increasing pile of bills out of my sight. He also didn't want to go out of the house without me, just in case I needed something. Tim was in desperate need of an outlet—something to open the relief valve and ease up on the pressure he had building up inside. I could hear his frustration when he spoke to his friends on the telephone. He was especially loud and vocal about his disdain for the treatment I was getting. Tim is passive-aggressive. That's an individual who expresses their negative feelings subtly through their actions instead of dealing with them directly. I kind of got the feeling he *wanted* me to hear these things but couldn't bring himself to say them directly to me. It was very disconcerting. I was afraid and wanted his help and input, but his disapproval made that almost impossible. This was uncharted territory for me. We had never had a major problem like this before. I didn't want to hurt him—not just because I *needed* him but because I am deeply and hopelessly in love with him. He is the last person I would want to hurt. I felt isolated and trapped and didn't know how to handle it.

When I was a teenager, I read the book *Joni* (pronounced Johnny), the true story of Joni Eareckson Tada, whom I mentioned earlier. In 1967, at only seventeen, she had a tragic swimming accident and became a quadriplegic. I suppose that since I was seventeen when I read the book, it hit close to home. Before she broke her neck, she had lived an active and athletic life. I imagined how hard it must have been for her to face the fact that she would never be able to walk again or do something as simple as roll over in bed. Reading the book changed my outlook on life. Although I read the book many years ago, there was something from her story that I remembered. She was frustrated and reluctant to accept that she was now crippled. Joni had to learn how to live with her disability and think outside of her suffering and consider others.

I was physically miserable, but I didn't want to be a miserable person. Even though I felt awful, I didn't want to deflect my frustration and anger onto anyone, especially Tim. I wanted him to know I appreciated his hard work, and I made sure I thanked him anytime he did something for me (even if it wasn't exactly what I wanted). I'll explain what I mean.

Tim loves sandwiches. I mean, he really loves to eat a *good* sandwich every day. His sandwiches, no matter what kind of lunchmeat he has in them, are topped with mayonnaise, lettuce, and tomato. Ham and cheese? Mayo, lettuce, and tomato. Liverwurst? Mayo, lettuce, and tomato. Bologna? Mayo, lettuce, and tomato. You get the idea. Now, I rarely eat sandwiches. I'm a bread snob. Unless the bread is really fresh, I won't eat it. The bread also has to be the kind I like. Don't even try to give me potato bread—*ugh!* A nice, freshly baked Portuguese roll is perfect. I put different condiments on my sandwiches too, depending on what's in it. Sometimes it's butter and mustard, sometimes it's mayo, sometimes it's oil and vinegar or nothing at all. This greatly perplexes Tim. He can't understand how anyone could eat a sandwich that doesn't have—you guessed it—mayo, lettuce, and tomato.

When I was unable to do much, he would prepare a midday meal for me. In his mind, there is only one thing to eat at noon, and that's a sandwich. If he made me a sandwich using hard bread and topped with mayo and a nasty, soggy tomato, I would smile, thank him, and eat it. I really was trying to be polite, but I needed some help and guidance. How should I approach him with this without insulting him and sounding ungrateful?

I thought it might be good to vent to someone about what I was experiencing (about everything, not just Tim's choice of lunch). Dr. Dawn recommended some counselors, but I wanted to speak with somebody who knew what I was going through—a survivor, not a professional. I decided to call the American Cancer Society. I took my phone and quietly went outside to make the call. I didn't want Tim to hear me. The woman on the other end of the line was very understanding. She thought it would be beneficial if I spoke with a breast cancer survivor.

These volunteers meet with you one on one and share their experiences, both good and bad, to help you through your journey. She also suggested I sign up for a class called "Look Good, Feel Better." This class, specifically for breast cancer patients, teaches tips and tricks to camouflage the lack of hair, dark circles under your eyes, and dry, irritated skin. Each woman who attends is given a case of cosmetics to help her look her best while she feels her worst. That sounded exactly like what I needed, so I agreed to both.

After the phone call, I found my own release from the pressure I was feeling and sat down to a *Star Wars* marathon. I normally had a hard time sitting through one movie, never mind four. It was uncharacteristic, but the force was with me that day as I allowed myself the luxury of doing something solely for me. Even then, in between light-saber duels and intergalactic dogfights, my mind jumped back to the present at light speed, and I got a knot in the pit of my stomach. Rosa was coming over today to cut my thinning hair. Like Tim, she's a *doer*, and she wanted to *do* something. I knew cutting my hair would help out both Tim and me.

Tim could cut my hair, but this was a difficult chore, and I didn't want to give him another burden to bear. You see, Tim loved my long hair. He derived so much pleasure from brushing it and braiding it. I must admit that I enjoyed the attention I got from him too. Had I not lost it all, his next step was to learn how to French braid. No, I didn't want Tim to cut my hair. It would have been too difficult for both of us. I presume it was hard for Rosa too, but she didn't show it. Knowing her, she probably cried in her car on the way home.

When Rosa arrived, we all went out on the back deck, and on this picture-perfect afternoon, she cut about seven inches off the bottom. This would be my last haircut for about two years. I took photos of the before and after. I began taking pictures of everything along the way. I'm not a particularly good photographer, but I thought it would be helpful to document this journey.

The following day was not an easy one. First, Tim and I had *words*. Let me interject here that we learned it was always good, in the long run, to talk and get everything off our chests, but it was not always easy. I've heard it said that sometimes the hardest thing and the right thing are the same thing. We both came to the realization that we needed to be brutally honest with each other but wrap it in love.

It's easy when you're married and are so familiar with each other that you forget just how precious your spouse is. One might lash out without ever giving it a second thought. A question I ask myself is, "How important is it?" Take the sandwich I mentioned earlier (please). The food on my plate might not have been my favorite thing to eat, but it's not *that* important. What I actually said, later on, when we were having a lighthearted conversation was, "Oh, by the way, I really appreciate that you made lunch for me, but maybe next time you could leave off the mayo and tomato." It sounds simple in principle, but it's not always easy to do. I'm human, so there were times when I wasn't so genteel. That was when Tim extended grace to me. Marriage isn't a fifty/fifty proposition, it's 100 percent/100 percent.

Speaking of sandwiches, at lunchtime the following day Tim made a *good* one and was just sitting down to eat. He had his back to me as I was perched on the truhe. I felt a large tangle in my hair, so I decided to get a pick and attempt to remove the knot. As I held the clump of hair in my right hand and gently worked on the snarl, I realized the hair I was holding was no longer attached to my head! By the time Tim finished eating and turned around to look at me, there was a huge pile of hair on the floor and hardly any on my head. There I sat, dumbfounded. I thought I had more time. I looked like I had mange. There was a mish-mash of wispy, dry, and frizzy hair on my head, interspersed with large bald spots. Now I *did* look like the Toxic Avenger.

As I stood in front of the mirror, I didn't recognize my reflection. I couldn't believe what I saw. I frantically went searching for scarves, a hat, *something—anything* to put over this mess on my head. Everything I tried on looked like I was trying to hide the fact that I hardly had any hair. We were going to the midweek service at church that evening, and I wasn't about to stay home and feel sorry for myself.

I found a bandana and played around with it, spreading what hair was left, here and there to make it appear that I wasn't balding. It didn't look great, but it had to do until I got my wig. I was glad that I hadn't waited until this point to order the wig. The woman at the center said most ladies who go there to be sized for their hairpiece already have lost all or most of their hair.

I felt like a '60s holdover, with a bandana and a denim jacket, but I held my head high and smiled as we walked into the sanctuary. It was a Wednesday night, when it's usually more casual, so I didn't stand out too much. Tim was playing, and he had to set up his equipment, so we were a little early. He desperately needed the diversion. Drumming is not only enjoyable for him, but it's also therapeutic. I brought my journal to pass the time before the service started. In truth, I was trying to stay by myself, act casual, and not draw any attention. However, after the service, as I sat in the pew, waiting for Tim, several ladies spontaneously came over to minister to me. They cheerfully greeted me (without the *look*) and asked if they could pray for me. It was wonderful. One woman anointed me with oil. Another told me, after I confided in her about my hair, that God had made only so many perfect heads, and on the rest, He put hair. Others quoted comforting scripture verses. They treated me with such sweet tenderness. One woman even told me that as she prayed, she got a sense of how much God loves me! I'm not sure if they will ever know, this side of heaven, what their thoughtfulness and prayers did for me that night. I was overwhelmed with joy.

That interaction was beautiful, but there were times when exchanges with some people resulted in a mental meltdown. It was extremely hard to control my emotions—another *wonderful* side effect of the chemo. Things that normally wouldn't upset me now caused great anxiety. It was as if my brain couldn't shut down, and I would replay negative conversations over and over in my head. I think I was still trying to deal with everything as if I were OK, and I wasn't. I didn't know how to handle this new reality. However, my oldest, Erin, came to my rescue and advised me to just not talk with anyone who upset me. She affirmed that I was going through a lot, and I needed to put me first. It was simple and exactly what I needed to hear. She was right. I was in an emotional upheaval, and I needed to set boundaries.

One thing I needed to do was get something beside a bandana to cover my head. I knew my wig would be in soon, but until then, I didn't want to walk around like this. I picked out a few gaiter-type scarfs. I had never seen anything like them before. I was thrilled that I could wear them in different ways, and they looked stylish. Once, I twisted it on the side and added a pretty silver pin. That did two things for me. It made me feel more feminine, and since it was my mother's pin, I felt close to her. I don't care how old you are, you never outgrow your need for your mommy. On one hand, I was glad she wasn't here to see me like this because it would have broken her heart. But on the other hand, I so desperately wanted to have her hold me and tell me everything was going to be OK. It was the second anniversary of her trip home to be with the Lord. I mourned but not for her. I mourned for me because I missed her so very much. There was no reason to grieve for her. Mom is now in the best place ever.

> For we know that if our earthly house, this tent, is destroyed, we have a building from God, a house not made with hands, eternal in the heavens. (2 Corinthians 5:1)

She is not sick anymore and doesn't need her hearing aids, glasses, and that cane that she detested so. No, the sadness was for me.

By now, I was virtually bald. I felt ugly. But I got some news that cheered me up a bit. My wig had arrived, and we had an appointment to get it. I also arranged to have the remainder of the sparse strands shaved off. This helps the wig to fit better and prevents random wisps from sticking out. The haircut was done in a private room. I was mortified to have anyone see me like this, but grateful I didn't have to go to a beauty parlor and sit for all the world to see. This was the one and only time I allowed Tim to see my naked head. I was so humiliated and prayed the whole time. It didn't take long but felt like forever. The technician was cognizant of my discomfort and turned the chair around so I didn't have to look in the mirror and watch as the last trace of my femininity was shorn off. Tim held my hand and made sure he smiled the whole time. He told me how beautiful I was and that I had a "perfectly shaped head." That made me laugh, but it's not the kind of compliment you ever want to hear from the love of your life.

The hair prosthesis came with all kinds of instructions—how to put it on; how to take it off; how to store it, wash it, and dry it. Also, what *not* to do, like go near open flames (no barbecues or marshmallow roasting), blow it dry, or brush it while it's wet. When we went outside into the real world, I felt like me. A delivery man was there, dropping off some packages, and I remember thinking, *I don't have to be ashamed to face people.* I was so happy and asked Tim take pictures, which I immediately sent to all my girls. It was the first time in a long while that I smiled, and it felt good.

During this time, I had stopped writing in my journal because I just didn't want to put pen to paper to record all the bad news. I had another chemo treatment and was not feeling great. I was nowhere as sick as the first time but sure didn't feel wonderful. Regardless of how I felt, after getting the wig, we had a visit to see Dr. Nett, and it was difficult. He told me that he thought he might have to perform a mastectomy after all. The masses were close to my nipple, and he thought a lumpectomy would leave me maimed. He proposed removing the entire breast and then reconstructing a new one. He said it was his opinion that this would be a better option, aesthetically, as I wouldn't be disfigured. He recommended a plastic surgeon he thought would do a fantastic job. This news was a lot to digest. I just wanted to run and hide. When I finally did start writing in my journal again, I wrote,

> Fear not, for I am with you; Be not dismayed, for I am your God. I will strengthen you, Yes, I will help you, I will uphold you with My righteous right hand. (Isaiah 41:10)

We had a busy schedule, and the day wasn't over yet. We were scheduled to go to the oncologist's office next. It was just a routine checkup, but I still didn't like going there.

Dr. Dawn didn't know I had lost all my hair, and as she examined me, she asked if I was going to get a wig. My new hair looked so natural and so *me* that she thought I still had my own hair but had cut it shorter. I was tickled pink.

When I went on disability, I wasn't just physically impaired; I was financially disabled as well. Weeks passed, and I had yet to see a check. The medical bills were coming in, and our regular expenses didn't stop just because I wasn't working. The rent, gas, electric, and health insurance still had to be paid, not to mention that we kind of liked eating too.

God is referred to by several names in the Bible. Each of these names has great significance and tells us something important about

Him. One of His names is Jehovah-Jireh,[20] which means "the Lord Will Provide." Instead of worrying about where our next meal was going to come from, I decided instead to trust that God would provide for us. His Word tells us to ask Him for what we need. So I did.

We were getting low on everything. I looked into the freezer and saw only one piece of meat left for dinner, and then that was it—just ice cubes. I said to Tim, "We still have food for one day, but don't worry, God will provide." And don't you know? He did just that! The following day, when our cupboards were bare, we got a message from church. It seemed that an anonymous donor had left us a generous gift card for the local supermarket.

This gift reminded me of manna. You've likely heard of superfoods; well, manna was the supernatural food that God gave to the Israelites while they were wandering in the desert. This amazing meal, which was said to "taste like wafers made with honey," was provided to them every day.

> And in the morning the dew lay all around the camp. And when the layer of dew lifted, there, on the surface of the wilderness, was a small round substance, as fine as frost on the ground. So when the children of Israel saw it, they said to one another, "What is it?" For they did not know what it was. (Exodus 16:13b–15)

They had never seen anything like it and didn't know what it was. I find it fascinating that they always had enough. They never went hungry, but they could not stockpile the manna. Each morning, for six days, the manna appeared. They were to gather what they needed for that day only. If anyone tried to save some for

---

[20] "And Abraham called the name of the place, The-LORD-Will-Provide; as it is said to this day, 'In the Mount of the LORD it shall be provided'" (Genesis 22:14).

the following day, they would find the manna had started to smell bad and was full of maggots. As no work was to be done on the Sabbath, however, twice as much manna could be collected on the sixth day. They were instructed to save some of it for the seventh day. Miraculously, that stored manna didn't go bad—no stink, no maggots. I felt like the gift card we had received came exactly when we needed it—not too early, not too late, just like manna.

Having cancer was like going to the school of hard knocks. During my education to get my degree in survival, I learned to *choose* to rely on the absolute assurance that God is sovereign and is in control of everything. In Matthew 10:29, we read about sparrows. This is a snippet of what Jesus told his disciples: "Are not two sparrows sold for a copper coin? And not one of them falls to the ground apart from your Father's will." (When I was in grammar school, I would buy candy like that—two gumballs for a penny.) But Jesus wasn't only telling them that God knows when a piddling little bird drops out of a tree. No, He was explaining God's sovereignty to them. Not only does our heavenly Father see the sparrow when it falls, but unless it is God's will, it cannot fall. I needed to remember that *nothing* happens without God's awareness and concern. When things seem to be going south for me, it is not an indicator that God has forgotten me.

In addition, God is so powerful; His Word says He holds everything together. "He is before all things, and in Him all things hold together" (Colossians 1:17). I reasoned that since He holds it all together, He certainly can protect and repair it. Therefore, I hypothesized, God could control the chemo as it was being pumped through my veins. Chemo is given to people with the intent of killing the cancerous cells. The chemo, however, doesn't know which cells are which, and it has the potential to damage your organs. I was concerned about my heart. It was strong and healthy, and I didn't like the thought of having this poison injected into it. So I prayed for the protection of my heart, kidneys, liver, skin, spleen, blood, and any other body part I could think of.

Another one of God's names is Jehovah-Rapha[21]—"the Lord Who Heals." I was confident that God could direct the chemo to go where it was supposed to go and destroy what it was supposed to destroy but leave the rest alone. One of my pastors encourages us to pray big. We say God is all powerful and mighty; shouldn't our prayers to Him reflect that? I say yes!

It's pretty cool that God has different names to describe His character. This might be a fun thing for us to adopt. I think a good second name for Rosa would be—*Lei Che Ti Nutre,* which is Italian for "She Who Feeds You." Every few days, she would call me. If I didn't answer, she'd contact Tim. She really wanted to *do* something to help, and since she's Italian, that help usually came in the form of something to eat. She thought it would be good medicine to go out to lunch. Very few things I ate tasted yummy, as my grandson says. Most everything had a metallic aftertaste, but I can tell you that the good medicine was getting out of the house and being with friends. I drove my car for the first time in two months, and it felt liberating. The scenery at the restaurant was delightful. Our table was on the patio in the warm sunshine, just feet from New Jersey's largest lake. I didn't realize that Rosa hadn't told our friend Marissa that I had cancer.

I felt awkward when she complimented me on my new hairdo. I didn't know what to say and just blurted out, "I have cancer. This is a wig." Poor Marissa. Her eyes welled up, and she had a look of horror on her face. I felt like such an idiot. I think I scared the woman half to death. I quickly followed up with, "But I'm OK!" She exhaled in relief. (Note to self: try to be a tad more sensitive around others when talking about cancer.)

That afternoon I felt *normal.* No one knew I was sick. I was just another face in the crowd, and I liked it that way. We talked and laughed. The girls even discussed taking a boat ride, but I had to bow out. I was too tired and afraid of getting seasick, as my tummy was already a little queasy. We said our goodbyes, and as I got into

---

[21] Exodus 15:22–26.

the car, I took a deep breath. I didn't think this simple lunch date would be so tiring. I was exhausted and couldn't wait to get home and pass out. I wrote the following in my journal:

> I know I feel weak, but no matter how I "feel," I need to, in my heart of hearts, believe in God's sovereignty and power and strength. I need to call on His name no matter how I feel! I need to *choose* to trust God.
>
> That we should no longer be children, tossed to and fro and carried about with every wind of doctrine, by the trickery of men, in the cunning craftiness of deceitful plotting. (Ephesians 4:14)
>
> So no matter how I "feel," I need to be firm in my belief that God is sovereign. He loves me, and I need to stick with my "know so" and not just be tossed about by my feelings.

When I mention *know so*, I'm referring to something I said during my mother's eulogy. I didn't want to talk about all the things she did or the kind of person she was because I felt that after ninety-five years, everyone already knew that. I wanted to talk about *why* she did what she did. I referenced Hebrews 11:1—"Now faith is the substance of things hoped for, the evidence of things not seen." I explained that my mother had a deep, abiding faith in God. Her hope wasn't an *I hope so*—hope, as in I *hope* my team wins the Super Bowl this year. No, her hope was an *I know so* hope. She knew her Savior was real and sovereign.

I watched her as she was dying. I saw her already slight frame waste away. Her body was starting to break down, and she knew her time was close at hand. She was never afraid, never complained, and never doubted God or His Word. This impressed me and gave me strength. This is where the rubber meets the road. This God she served was real, and she knew it. She had confidence in what she didn't see.

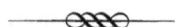

It would still be about four months before I had surgery, but Dr. Nett thought it was a good idea for me to meet the plastic surgeon. I took this option for granted, but prior to 1998, when a woman faced having a mastectomy, reconstruction was, many times, out of the question. Insurance companies usually didn't cover the costs, as it was considered cosmetic. The average woman couldn't afford to spend hundreds of thousands of dollars for reconstruction. Then, the Women's Health and Cancer Rights Act of 1998[22] was enacted, which provided protections to patients who chose to have breast reconstruction. It stated that if you received benefits in connection with a mastectomy, and you elected breast reconstruction, coverage must be provided for the following:

- All stages of reconstruction of the breast on which the mastectomy was performed
- Surgery and reconstruction of the other breast to produce a symmetrical appearance
- Prostheses and treatment of physical complications of all stages of the mastectomy, including lymphedema

I have become more grateful that the medical community has realized breast reconstruction is vitally important to healing from breast cancer.

Dr. Nett highly recommended Dr. Nòvel, and I'm forever grateful that he did. My appointment to see the plastic surgeon was

---

[22] "Women's Health and Cancer Rights Act of 1998," 437–439, https://www.govinfo.gov/content/pkg/PLAW-105publ277/pdf/PLAW-105publ277.pdf.

during the middle of morning rush hour, and, as a result, the stop-and-go driving nauseated me. I was frustrated and was green behind the gills when I met the doctor for the first time. I wanted to be fresh and alert so I could ask questions and listen intently to everything he had to say. This was a big deal for me. I tried to be totally prepared. I even brought all my medications with me so I could fill out the patient information form correctly. There were so many pills—a yellow one for nausea, larger pills in a blister pack for severe nausea, blue ones taken prior to chemo, a white one for anxiety, antibiotics for an infection; you get the idea.

I was nervous and felt intimidated to meet a plastic surgeon. I'm not an elegant-looking woman. I don't have fancy jewelry or wear expensive clothes. This was way out of my comfort zone. I was sure that as an upscale plastic surgeon, he got many patients with large Prada pocketbooks who wanted all kinds of body-enhancing procedures. In contrast, I was plain Jane from the country, who just didn't fit in. I wasn't seeking to augment my bust size; I just wanted to be put back together after the mastectomy and be *me* again.

The doctor's appearance, however, did fit the ideal of what you'd imagine a plastic surgeon would resemble. He wore a trendy and (I'm sure) overpriced suit with stylish leather shoes. There was nothing off-the-rack about this man. His hair was perfectly coiffed, with enough gray blended in to give his youthful face a distinguished look of experience. His sparkling dark eyes appeared to smile at me with an air of confidence and say, "Everything is going to be all right." His perfect skin was the color of a gourmet latte, and his teeth were as white as the foam on top of that latte. In other words, Dr. Nòvel was the real-life version of Dr. McDreamy.

I was expecting a no-nonsense, time-is-money kind of guy, but that wasn't the case. He was empathetic and gentle, and he listened intently to everything I had to say. Dr. Nòvel was aware that what he was telling me was a lot to process, and he reassured me that he would explain everything to me, step by step, when the time came.

At this point, I was convinced I would have a bilateral

mastectomy and would use a combination of my own fat and implants to reconstruct my breasts. I was aware that all this meant at least three operations. I wasn't looking forward to it, but I wanted *me* back. I didn't want the scars of cancer to be the first thing I noticed when I saw my reflection. I knew the decisions I made now would affect me for the rest of my life. I also knew that some of these decisions would be easy to make but hard to do. I love my Tim, but the reconstruction was for me. I was learning to hear my own voice and realized I could trust God to guide me.

Chapter 7

I'M NOT JUST LEARNING HOW TO SURVIVE BUT HOW TO LIVE

No matter what changes come or the turmoil I face, I find great security in the fact that my God is steadfast. People change their minds all the time, and fads are short-lived. Remember pet rocks? How about fidget spinners? What's hot today is passé tomorrow. In contrast, I can depend on God. He doesn't change with the times.

What *did* change was how my body reacted to each chemo treatment. We called it the symptom du jour. We never knew what to expect. Some weeks, I was exhausted and slept both night and day. Other times, I was weepy and emotional, or had diarrhea, or was constipated, or my skin was dry and itchy, or I had restless legs, or my belly was so bloated I looked pregnant. You name it. Just about everything tasted yucky, but that varied as well. At one point, my mouth had such a chemical reaction to orange juice that I thought I was ingesting battery acid. It burned my mouth, and I quickly chased it down with a cold glass of water. Once, I made potato salad, and it was delicious. I couldn't wait to get home from the doctor and have some for lunch. After the treatment, however, the salad tasted like it had somehow gone rotten in that short time. Only three food items always appealed to me: peaches, yogurt, and shrimp (not all at once, mind you). Although I wasn't too enthusiastic about eating, I still managed to get heavier. (What's up with that?) I thought for sure I would shed a few pounds, but no. Am I the only one who gets cancer and *gains* weight? Little did I know that it was a very good thing I did. I would need that extra fat around my midsection to help reconstruct my new breast.

Speaking of side effects, I wasn't the only one being affected. Tim would sometimes exhibit the same symptoms I did. The more I researched, the more I saw that this phenomenon is not unusual. Caregivers frequently feel that they too are going through the pain, just like you. In addition, according to a study[23] I read, they also feel frustrated, angry, drained, guilty, or helpless, although they may not let on. If you think you were ill-prepared to get the diagnosis of cancer, just think of how the caregiver feels. Most, if not all, of the support goes to the patient. It is expected that the spouse, child, or friend will become the caregiver, but they are thrown into this role with little or no support. I was sick; that took no special skill on my part. Tim was doing all the work. He was giving everything he had to help me, and there was nothing left for himself. I encouraged him to join a men's Bible study, if only to get out of the house (away from me) and be with his peers. He took my advice and, as of this writing, is still studying God's Word with these men who have become his close friends. Ecclesiastes 4:9–10 confirms that it is good to have companionship: "Two are better than one, Because they have a good reward for their labor. For if they fall, one will lift up his companion. But woe to him who is alone when he falls, For he has no one to help him up." If you are reading this and there is a devoted person in your

---

[23] M. Pinquart and S. Sorensen, "Differences between Caregivers and Noncaregivers in Psychological Health and Physical Health: A Meta-Analysis," *Psychology and Aging* 18, no. 2 (2003): 250–267.

life caring for you, do something to make sure he or she gets breaks, has a support system, and receives training on *how* to care for others.

To help myself, I spoke with Mrs. Verde, the volunteer from the American Cancer Society. She was a twenty-year survivor of breast cancer. I found our talks encouraging, and I enjoyed speaking with her. We were both diagnosed with invasive ductal carcinoma. Mrs. Verde described her treatment and how she dealt with it. I was aghast, however, when I realized we had the same protocol. She had been diagnosed two decades earlier, yet our protocols were identical. I couldn't believe that after twenty years, in this age of advanced technology and millions of dollars donated for research, that there wasn't an iota of difference in our care. This discouraged me greatly. Was there a cure out there, but because of the huge influx of money, *they* (whoever *they* are) didn't want to kill the goose that laid the golden egg? Or was it just because this treatment worked so *if it ain't broke, don't fix it*?

This wasn't something I wanted to hear. Now, I wanted to become a doer and not so passive with my care. I wasn't about to stop the traditional treatment I was receiving, but I certainly was open to trying additional therapies to move along the process of destroying this cancer. Again, I *always* recommend to anyone who contemplates this to discuss it with their medical professionals *first*.

After reviewing it with Dr. Dawn, I began to assist her with my care. I was already taking comprehensive vitamin and mineral supplements, but I continued adding things that might help.

Tim was diving into research on alternative ways to treat cancer. Although discouraged, I wasn't about to ditch the conventional care I was getting because that gave me the best odds of beating cancer. I read articles and watched videos of folks who rejected any kind of traditional treatment and instead used salves, exercise, certain foods, and vitamins *alone* to battle their various types of cancer. Sadly, their homegrown cures didn't achieve the desired outcome, and they succumbed to the cancer. Nonetheless, I was extremely interested in finding ways to *assist* the doctors to eradicate this nasty disease from my body. Tim bought books written by naturopathic medical doctors who treated their patients using integrative oncology. In short, *integrative oncology* is an evidence-based specialty that combines naturopathic (natural remedies) therapies with traditional medical treatment.[24] Tim also watched a series of videos that discussed studies from around the world. They hit on topics such as chemotherapy, cancer facts and fictions, viruses, different things that cause and fuel cancer, detoxing, and much more.

One way to be proactive in my fight against cancer and not just a bystander was to change my eating habits. I reasoned that enhancing my body's own immune system couldn't hurt. The first item that bit the dust was aspartame. This artificial sweetener is controversial. The FDA says it is safe, while other sources say it is not. I preferred to err on the side of caution and deep-sixed it. I heard that cancer likes sugar. Again, there are studies that concur with this thought and others that disagree. I chose to limit my intake of sugar, as a precaution.

Some of the things I added to my menu were organic olive oil, flaxseed, and honey. And even though I already liked and ate blueberries, peaches, spinach, olives, broccoli, garlic, brussels sprouts, and unflavored yogurt, I loaded up on these foods. Water isn't my favorite beverage, but I made sure I stayed hydrated and avoided caffeine. Like a majority of Americans, I enjoy a good cup of joe. Regrettably, though, the chemo made even the aroma of coffee so repulsive that I was unable to drink any at all. What I did enjoy was Melaleuca tea. This herbal tea is a blend of Melaleuca alternifolia leaves, cinnamon, and chamomile flower. I tried taking turmeric, but the chemo made this a hard pill to swallow (pun intended).

In Tim's research on healthy eating, we found that blood oranges are rich in antioxidants. Antioxidants are nutrients and enzymes that fight free radicals that can cause cancer or do damage to our blood

---

[24] S. M. Sagar, "Integrative oncology in North America," *J Soc Integr Oncol*. 41 (2006): 27–39. Google ScholarPubMed

vessels and organs. The concept of free radicals may be hard to grasp, but in layman's terms, here goes my attempt at explaining it. Electrons like to be in pairs. Free radicals are single atoms that forage through the body, looking for other electrons so they can become a pair. While they are rooting around in there, looking for a mate, they can damage your body.

All this new information was overtaxing my chemo brain! Tim was doing so much research and trying to fill my head with this wonderful new knowledge, but I was having trouble remembering how to spell my name. He'd been used to me being a tough bird, but at this point, I was more like a tender chicken.

I mentioned an herbal tea we enjoy called Melaleuca—Tim and I have been using this and many other products from a company by the same name. During this journey, I personally found these natural-based products to be greatly beneficial. Most of the effects of the chemo, so far (minus losing my hair), were on the inside of my body. However, other problems started to crop up on the outside. My skin was dry and itchy; I was getting fever blisters and sores on my arms and in my mouth. It also hurt to pee. So using Melaleuca's intensive skin lotion, lip balm, and supplements greatly helped.

Tim has benefited from Melaleuca's vitamin and mineral supplements for decades and, as a result, has maintained good health, both inside and out. These supplements aren't your run-of-the-mill, one-a-day supplements that you buy at the supermarket. These vitamins have a unique triple-patented absorption property. This means that when you take a typical supplement, your body has difficulty absorbing them into your system. The process Melaleuca's supplements use, called Oligo,[25] keeps minerals soluble and available for absorption so they can more easily pass through your intestinal wall and benefit your body. I reasoned that if I was going to spend

---

[25] Melaleuca, "Mounting Evidence Confirms Oligo's Superior Antioxidant Protection," April 30, 2010, https://www.melaleuca.com/Oligo/Content.aspx?Page=SuperiorScience.

the time and money on supplements, I might as well get the ones that gave me the most benefit. I'm not saying that this company is the only one to provide a safe and natural way to achieve good health and stay that way. I just thought it would be a good idea to explain what we did that proved to be beneficial to us. As always, do your own research and talk to your doctors.

Another good way to live a healthy lifestyle is to limit your exposure to harmful elements. My Tim is serious about cleaning. He's also serious about avoiding toxins, so we use safe, natural cleaning products, also from Melaleuca. Some people may not be aware that many everyday cleaning products are more harmful to our health than we might imagine. The results of a twenty-year independent study published in the *American Journal of Respiratory and Critical Care Medicine*[26] showed:

- Using national-brand cleaners as little as once per week is as damaging to lung health as smoking twenty cigarettes per day.
- Cleaning at home is just as harmful, if not more so, than being an occupational cleaner.
- Women who regularly use cleaning products have increased rates of asthma.
- Damage is cumulative over time.
- Cleaning products can irritate the eyes or throat or cause headaches and other health problems, including cancer.

---

[26] Ø Svanes, RJ Bertelsen, SHL Lygre, AE Carsin, JM Antó, B Forsberg, JM García-García, JA Gullón, J Heinrich, M Holm, M Kogevinas, I Urrutia, B Leynaert, JM Moratalla, N Le Moual, T Lytras, D Norbäck, D Nowak, M Olivieri, I Pin, N Probst-Hensch, V Schlünssen, T Sigsgaard, TD Skorge, S Villani, D Jarvis, JP Zock and C Svanes, "Cleaning at home and at work in relation to lung function decline and airway obstruction," June 19, 2007, https://doi.org/10.1164/rccm.200612-1793OC, and https://www.thoracic.org/about/newsroom/press-releases/resources/women-cleaners-lung-function.pdf
American Lung Association, July 13, 2020, https://www.lung.org/clean-air/at-home/indoor-air-pollutants/cleaning-supplies-household-chem.

Knowing what I now know about cancer, these findings are eye-opening. I became aware that being healthy is a way of life and much more than just walking around the block once a day and avoiding carbonated beverages. Again, I stress that anything you do outside of your normal protocol should be discussed with your doctor(s). I did this ad nauseam. Although Dr. Dawn was a by-the-book type of doctor, if it didn't interfere with her traditional treatment, she didn't balk; surprisingly, she was knowledgeable about everything I mentioned to her.

Even though I got along well with Dr. Dawn, going to the oncologist didn't get any easier. I'd enter the office a nervous wreck and make jokes to ease the stress, but there was no hiding that I was afraid and panicky. It was hard to focus on anything specific for too long, due to the haze that would envelope me. At times, it was physically difficult to even write in my journal while I was there, as my hands trembled. The shaking was caused by a combination of being cold, scared, and sick. I love gospel music and listening to that helped chase away my fear. (Listen to Hezekiah Walker's "Every Praise," and I'll be a monkey's uncle if your heart is not refreshed.) Again, kind words, prayers, and thoughtful gestures really helped. My prayer partners sent messages to encourage me. Juliet, my youngest, texted that she was praying for me, and that made all the difference that day.

We knew we couldn't escape the reality that I was sick, and we were in financial trouble. We did try, however, to do things to help us get some sort of respite from the doom and gloom of cancer treatment. Once a week during the summer months, a nearby town hosted "Music in the Park," where local bands played in a beautiful setting overlooking a lake. We are blessed in this area of the state to have a plethora of lakes. There are fourteen just in my little township alone. So every Friday after dinner, I would put on my wig and don something pretty and summery, as Tim gathered up the folding chairs, bug spray (natural, of course), and bottled water. For two hours, I wasn't sick, and Tim wasn't tired; we were just another couple, sitting on the grass, holding hands, enjoying the harmonies and melodies of country, blues, and rock 'n' roll.

It wasn't always easy to *do* things because I tired easily, but we tried to get a walk in whenever we could. There's an old train bed nearby that offers a perfect scenic walking path. As we strolled under the canopy of trees, we talked about anything and everything (except cancer). There were many hellos and how-are-yous as we passed entire families on bikes, runners preparing for the next race, and couples meandering, hand in hand, down the path. I knew Tim despised taking walks, but I also knew he loved me with all that was within him, and if this made me feel better, he was all in. How can you feel sad or depressed when someone does that for you?

A wonderful event we were both looking forward to was the birth of grandson number two. My Erin was glowing, the picture-perfect image of an expectant mother. She was going to have a baby shower, and I offered to make the favors, which were chocolate lollipops. This was a lot of work, but it did two things: got my mind off of how miserable I felt and made me happy to think about the little bundle that was on the way. I don't mind saying that I was tired, but it was curative. I finally felt like I was useful. Everyone else though it quite acceptable that I should put my feet up and chill out but doing so made me feel sluggish and lazy. It's easy to sit down and rest a spell, but it's not so simple to put your mind in timeout.

Chapter 8

J.O.Y. = JESUS, OTHERS, YOU

When I am tired, weak, and exceptionally bored, I look for things to keep my mind occupied. Popcorn projects were perfect. I call them that because I didn't have to spend a lot of time on them and could do them in spurts, like kernels of popcorn, bursting with energy a little at a time. Writing out thank-you notes to those who had blessed me was a perfect popcorn project. A maxim by William Arthur Ward describes my sentiment best: "Feeling gratitude and not expressing it is like wrapping a present and not giving it." I wanted the people in my life to know just how much I appreciated them and that their gestures comforted me. It might have been a kind word, a gift of a meal, a prayer, or just plain concern and thoughtfulness. Along with these notes, I included a Bible verse, a homemade chocolate lollipop, and a small gift. Some, like all the elders in our church, received a pen that had "SALVATION ... He nailed it!" written on it. Hidden inside was a scroll that read:

> Each worry, stress or sorrow,
> Each need you're thinking of …

> Nail it to the cross,
> And entrust it to Christ's love.
> A trial or temptation,
> A challenge hard to face ...
> Nail it to the cross,
> And give it to His grace.
> For Christ redeemed all suffering,
> All struggle, loss and death ...
> He "nailed" the world's salvation,
> As He took His final breath.

Others received a small keychain with either Psalm 46:1b on it—"God is our refuge and strength, A very present help in trouble"—or a part of John 15:12, which read, "Love one another." I prayed for each person as I wrote out these notes. This kept me busy and productive, and it had a wonderful side effect—I was being blessed too.

Bad habits come quite easily. Good habits, not so much. I made a conscious decision to incorporate some good habits into my daily routine. I increased my prayer time and lifted up all those who had surrounded me and cared for me, although they weren't the only ones I prayed for. I included those with whom I had strained relationships too. Again, I was the one being blessed.

Since I knew what a wonderful godsend it was to have sweet souls praying for me while I was sick, I began to concern myself and pray for those in my life who were ill. Sadly, several people I knew had gotten the dreaded cancer diagnosis. I received word that my dear friend Louisa, who lives in Texas, had endometrial cancer, a form of uterine cancer. This upset me, as I wanted to help her. I knew how hard it was for me, and I had Tim. I couldn't imagine how difficult it would be to go through this alone. Who would bring her to the hospital? Was there anyone who could help care for her after surgery? Would she be able to get to the store for food? I wished that I was well so I could travel there and help ease her burdens. But I couldn't, and that frustrated me. At the same time, two close friends from church were diagnosed with cancer: Sally with breast cancer and Foster with lymphoma. In addition, a young man I worked with discovered he had cancerous tumors on his kidneys, and my brother-in-law had a brain tumor. I knew how bad this disease was treating me, and I empathized greatly with each of these precious people.

When I saw Foster for the first time after hearing of his diagnosis, I couldn't help but cry. It was sad to see someone so full of life and joy, so kind and thoughtful, get hit with this nasty illness. Well, Foster would have none of that, and he began to encourage me. Whenever I bumped into him (and even now, years later), Foster would tell me that he prayed for me every day. He was (and is) such an encouragement and inspiration. His face never lacked a smile, and he gave God all the glory. That's how I wanted to be, but I'm afraid I fell far short of that goal.

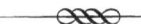

I was going to go to the Look Good, Feel Better class. I was excited, but I felt bad that we had to travel about an hour away, and Tim couldn't come in. The class was for breast cancer patients only. The ladies leading the class were empathetic to the patients' mental states and knew that having a third party there could be embarrassing for some. Tim shrugged it off as no big deal.

The class was held in the breast cancer wing of a hospital. I wasn't sure what to expect, but after the women started arriving, I felt quite comfortable. These ladies were me. One woman was bald and wore a baseball cap. Another showed up with a scarf on her head. I think I was the only one there with a wig. After we were all shepherded into a room, we were given a large maroon (Yay! Not pink!) case filled with makeup and supplies. The cosmetics weren't identical, as they were donated. My case held nail polish, foundation, eyebrow pencil, eyeliner, lip liner and lipstick, rouge, mascara, and all sorts of brushes to apply the cosmetics. Some women additionally received sunblock, and skin moisturizer. It was like getting an early birthday present.

There were eight of us, plus the esthetician (one trained to administer facials and advise on makeup and the care of skin and hair) and the instructor, sitting around the table, when the door burst open, and a loud woman came in with a man. She spoke with a thick accent and apologized for being late. The teacher politely explained that the class was just for patients. The lady, whom I shall call Annika, said she didn't speak English well, and this was her interpreter. She gestured toward a young man about twenty years old. He looked like he had just gotten out of bed. The hood of his sweatshirt was pulled up over his head, and his attention was focused on his cell phone.

Annika took a seat, and her interpreter slouched onto a chair behind her. I was not happy, nor was I comfortable. The teacher then asked the class if any of us minded if he was there. Everyone there said no, except for me. Tim would say I was being difficult, but I viewed it differently. Annika spoke English quite well, and I was not convinced she needed any help to communicate her thoughts. As a matter of fact, as I look back at that day, I don't remember ever hearing her interpreter say one word. The teacher explained that he could wait outside while we had the class, and Mr. Interpreter was all too ready to comply. I don't think he was too keen on spending two hours in a room crowded with a gaggle of bald women.

After the commotion settled down, we started the class. The teacher explained the history of Look Good, Feel Better and why she loved working with breast cancer patients. The Look Good, Feel Better philosophy is simple; they are dedicated to improving cancer patients' quality of life and self-esteem by offering free classes that teach beauty techniques to enable them to face their diagnoses with greater confidence.

Next, the esthetician had us go through all our products. One by one, she explained how to use each item to enhance our beauty or hide flaws, like creating eyebrows where there were none or how to conceal blotchy skin. Throughout the entire class, Annika, who was sitting two seats away from me, talked and laughed about everything. She really was a fun-loving person who had us all laughing.

The American Cancer Society provides wigs to cancer patients, and the woman in the baseball cap was getting hers that day. She was so thrilled when she put it on and looked in the mirror. She beamed as if she had won a million-dollar lottery. I learned later that until that day, she had been unable to wear a wig, as she had painful sores on her head. Another woman said her hair had not totally fallen out so she still had strands of her original hair. This hair, however, was brittle, and as her new hair grew back, she was afraid to brush the old hair for fear it would fall out and leave a bald spot.

I'm a talker, and when I get in a group of like-minded people, you can't shut me up. But that day, I was quiet and listened. My heart was overcome with gratitude. I started to witness firsthand how I was being protected from so many of the adverse effects of the chemo. I know that some of the precautions I took helped—for instance, applying an intensive skin-therapy lotion to my scalp probably aided in preventing sores—but I know, ultimately, God's hand was protecting me.

Next, we learned different ways to fashion a scarf and how to transform an inexpensive XXL T-shirt into a stylish head covering. There was a short video by Stacy London of the *What Not to Wear* television program. In it, Stacy instructed us how to use flattering colors and shapes of clothing to help camouflage areas of concern (e.g., no reconstruction, weight gain or loss). Next, we heard all about wigs and what to look for when selecting one, how to care for it, and what they cost. Everyone there was quite shocked to learn that my *hair* was a wig. That made my day.

By the time the class was over, we all looked beautiful. Our cheeks were rosy and so were our dispositions. We had come in quiet and timid, except for Annika, but left smiling and laughing. As we packed up our treasures, Annika stuffed her case with everything on the table, thinking they were all take-home items. When she was told otherwise, she laughed at her faux pas, took them out of her bag, and bounced out of the room. She provided much-needed comic relief to a tense atmosphere. No matter where you go in life, may you always have an Annika.

When I left the hospital, I was shining as brightly as the noonday sun. Tim peered out from the car window and could see, just by the glow on my face, that the class had been a positive experience. He too was happy and bursting at the seams to tell me about his day. As it turned out, we were not too far from his childhood home, so he decided to take a ride over and check out the old neighborhood. When he drove past his former home, he spied an old friend. The two spent the next hour sipping iced tea, reminiscing about old times, and catching up on current happenings. The day was such a delight. We both got exactly what we needed to lift our spirits.

I had been sick only about three months, but I was tired and bored and starting to get depressed. I couldn't imagine how it must feel to be unhealthy for years. My diagnosis wasn't that bad, and I had the hope of being well again. A few years ago, right before Tim and I got married, a vibrant young woman at church got colon cancer. She wound up in hospice because she needed the acute care. This precious soul was there for four years before she died, leaving behind two school-aged children and a husband.

I think of Joni Eareckson Tada, who never fully recovered from her injury. The apostle Paul spoke of his thorn in the flesh[27] that looks to have affected him for years. Have you ever heard of Nick Vujicic? This amazing man was born without arms or legs. When he was only ten years old, he tried to kill himself. By thirteen, he realized he had a choice to make: either be angry for what he didn't have or thankful for what he did have. He sought God and thought the Lord would heal him. Although he didn't get that miracle, he did get a purpose for his life when he met a little boy who also had been born without limbs. Nick saw how his story of courage and

---

[27] 2 Corinthians 12: 7–9.

perseverance encouraged the boy, and he thought it could also help others. He came to this realization: "When I don't get a miracle, I can still be a miracle for someone else."

I had absolutely no room to complain. My problems were miniscule compared to the ones these wonderful people endured. I had to *choose* to hope in the Lord. I needed to purposefully and willfully, no matter what my situation, live a life of gratitude to God.

God has a way of bringing a message to you again and again, until, hopefully, you get it. The big idea in the church service that week was that even when life seems out of control, Christ still calls the shots. Again, using my journal to organize my thoughts, document my journey, and encourage myself, I wrote the following:

> I need to turn down the noise and ask God what He wants to teach me.
> "being confident of this very thing, that He who has begun a good work in you will complete it until the day of Jesus Christ" (Philippians 1:6).

God is in control. His plans for me are good, and He will finish what He started. A dear friend of mine always quotes Jeremiah 29:11—"For I know the thoughts that I think toward you, says the LORD, thoughts of peace and not of evil, to give you a future and a hope." Also, Romans 15:13 says, "Now may the God of hope fill you with all joy and peace in believing, that you may abound in hope by the power of the Holy Spirit." To abound means to have so much that it overflows. Logically, if my hope is overflowing, it's flowing *somewhere*. I would like to think that hope is overflowing onto others and blessing them.

Chapter 9

EXPECT THE UNEXPECTED

I'm certain that God has quite a sense of humor. My head was as smooth as a baby's bottom; I had no eyebrows or eyelashes; and my arms were devoid of any hair. My legs were also bare—except below my knees. When I noticed this, I laughed heartily!

I read a devotional that said God is happy. In John 15:11, Jesus said, "These things I have spoken to you, that My joy may remain in you, and that your joy may be full." He has joy! And in 1 Timothy 1:11, the apostle Paul wrote, "According to the glorious gospel of the blessed God which was committed to my trust." Blessed means happy. I like that. I've never specifically thought about God being happy. Sometimes I think that we picture God sitting on His throne with a bunch of lightning bolts, just waiting for us to mess up so He can zap us.

To the contrary, in Matthew 25:23, Jesus is teaching about His return through the parable of the talents. In this story, a servant is rewarded for his faithfulness. It reads, "His lord said to him, 'Well done, good and faithful servant; you have been faithful over a few things, I will make you ruler over many things. Enter into the joy of your lord.'" And in Nehemiah 8:10b, we read, "for the joy of the LORD is your strength." He wants us to share in His joy! We usually think about God's judgment and skip over the joy part.

I wanted to be happy. Not too many *happy* things happen when you are in the throes of your cancer treatment, although there was one pleasant occurrence that I think was an anomaly. My fingernails and toenails grew in quick and strong. Nail changes are common during chemotherapy, but I've yet to read anything that says, "Oh, and by the way, periodically, chemo fortifies your nails." On the contrary, they get weak and brittle and can change shape. A fellow at work had rectal cancer, and he said all his fingernails turned black when he was in active treatment. Cancer patients who undergo chemo treatment may even lose their nails altogether. Fortunately, I hear this is less common, and I was thrilled that it didn't happen to me. As I've said, I asked Dr. Dawn many questions, including, "What is causing my fingernails to grow so beautifully?" I never did get a definitive answer, as the office said they hadn't heard of that happening before.

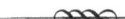

It was time for the baby shower. I would get to see all my children, including Tim's daughter, Rebecca. Blaise joined the other boys, both young and old, for a hike and then lunch, while all the ladies celebrated River's approaching appearance. I hadn't seen some of the people there since I was diagnosed and was a little timid about my looks. Thankfully, I blended right in and felt like one of the crowd.

The setting of the shower was beautiful. Café tables with bouquets of purple and blue hydrangeas in mason jars dotted the backyard around the in-ground pool. I sat on the deck that looked out over the yard, underneath an oversized patio umbrella. It was wonderful to watch the children splash about in the water. Everyone was smiling, and I was thrilled to be around my daughters. My taste buds were pleasantly surprised by the yumminess of the food. It was wonderful to celebrate life, as opposed to being surrounded by death and pain.

Juliet and Blaise stayed the night at our house before returning home the next day. She and Tim were busy doing laundry, which left Blaise and me with some alone time. His mommy had told him I was sick, but he wasn't sure what was going on. He studied my face whenever I talked to him, and I could tell the wheels were turning. It had been a long and tiring day, so to help Blaise wind down, we got comfortable with some blankets and pillows in front of the television. He wanted to watch *Star Wars*—again. After the droids spirited away the plans to the *Death Star* from the evil Empire in an escape pod, Blaise sat up and turned to look at me with a profoundly serious expression. "Nina, tell me the truth about why you are sick," he said. (I'm *Nina* because he couldn't say Nana when he was younger.)

It caught me by surprise and led me to believe he was much more perceptive than you'd expect from a five-year-old. His question demanded an honest answer. So I gave him one. "I have something called cancer."

I guess he had never heard of that before. "Cancer?" he asked.

"Yes, but I'm going to be better." I didn't want him to be worried.

"Will you be better in two days?" he queried.

"More like one hundred days."

"Wow, that's a lot," he said, squishing his eyebrows together. He pondered the new information I had given him, seemed satisfied with the answer, and returned his gaze to the screen to see 3PO and R2 trudge through the sands of Tatooine, on their quest to find Obi-Wan Kenobi.

The following morning, I talked to Blaise about my appearance. I hadn't seen him since Mother's Day, which was before any chemo treatments. The last time he saw me, my hair was down to the middle of my back. I explained that I was taking medicine to get well, but it had some side effects. I explained that I had lost all my hair, and I was wearing a wig. I didn't expose my bare head to him, but I did show him the wig and let him examine it. I could tell he was absorbing everything I said but didn't know what to do with the information. It made him visibly uncomfortable to see me with a scarf on my head, knowing I was bald, and he asked me to please put the wig back on.

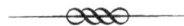

The optimism I had at the start of this journey had waned, but in its place, I had a strong and peaceful resolve. I expected Murphy's law: "Anything that can go wrong will go wrong and at the worst possible time." I also didn't get my hopes up, waiting for unicorns and rainbows to appear. Writer J. R. R. Tolkien, author of *Lord of the Rings*, said it best: "It does not do to leave a live dragon out of your calculations, if you live near him." Despite that, I was keenly aware that even in the chaos and pain of all that was happening, I was going to be all right because I knew *Who* was in control.

One tidbit of truth I garnered about oncologists is that the patient is on a need-to-know basis. They don't withhold information from you but only tell you what you need to know, when you need to know it, and nothing more. There were times when I had to pull all the particulars out of Dr. Dawn. I suspect she didn't want to overwhelm me with the entirety of my treatment. If patients got the whole scoop up front, they'd probably panic and feel like they couldn't possibly handle it all.

Here's how it usually went between Dr. Dawn and me: She would advise me of a protocol and tell me about how long it would take. Next, I'd think, *Great, I can handle this*. When this was completed, she'd then tell me that *we'd* be taking this new medicine for another X number of weeks. (Doctors tend to say *we*, but it was always *me*.) This back-and-forth protocol tango went on the entire time. It seemed as if I was never going to be done. I think, in oncology school, they tell future doctors that patients are scared and don't want to know, and I suppose this is true a majority of the time. I saw several bedraggled patients in the office who came in, took their blows, no questions asked, and smiled through the suffering because this was their salvation. I met one woman who was on a type of chemo for seven years. She was in a perpetual state of misery, but she nonetheless didn't question her treatment plan, because as far as she was concerned this was her lifeline. I, however, did not find comfort in the liquids flowing through the IV. The cancer didn't scare me as much as the chemo did.

Once again, I had the wind knocked out of my sails when Dr. Dawn advised me that my treatments wouldn't be over until the first week of September. Erin was expected to deliver her son at the beginning of October. I wanted to be healthy enough to see and hold my new grandbaby. *Sigh*. As Tom Petty said, "The waiting is the hardest part."

My journal for the next month and a half reflected the struggle of convalescing. Boober Fraggle once said, "Tedium and drudgery are good for the soul." However, being a Muppet, I'm sure he never experienced the stuff. Don't get me wrong; it was wonderful to be home, as I could not have managed working at my physically demanding job, but it was monotonous. It's also hard to relax when I hadn't gotten a paycheck in months. Our family members helped us out many times by providing meals and, from time to time, money to keep the bill collectors at bay. I wrote Proverbs 17:17 in my journal: "A friend loves at all times, And a brother is born for adversity."

A huge godsend was a fund we have at work. It is specifically there to aid employees who are going through financial difficulties. The associates donate money throughout the year, either through fundraisers, such as a cupcake sale or pancake breakfast, and/or by designating a mere dollar out of their paychecks every pay period, which the company then matches. It was the generosity of others via this fund that enabled us to pay the rent for three months. Once again, Jehovah-Jireh had delivered!

My entertainment during the summer was the flora and fauna around our home. The irises, hydrangeas, and azaleas were just breathtaking that year. The birdsong filled the air like a feathered choir. Watching swans, geese, and ducks on the lake, as a party boat lazily floated by, was so much better than sitting in front of the boob tube. Unfortunately, many days were also spent on the telephone, waiting for a representative from the state disability, a doctor's office, or an insurance company, while Muzak played. The only interruption to the incessant canned melody was a robotic voice chiming in every few minutes saying, "Your call is very important to us. Please hold until the next representative is available." I remember some calls on which I waited on hold for twenty minutes, only to be cut off. When I redialed the number, I got the recording: "All lines are currently busy. Please try again later."

Some calls had me press this button for *that*, press that button for *this*, and then I ended up with a prompt that had nothing to do with the reason I'd called. If you've ever gotten stuck in a recording loop while trying to get answers, you know what I mean. There were times when I yelled at the phone, "I want to speak with a human being!" and then hung up. That's one thing about landlines that are great—you can slam the receiver down on the base of the phone. It's hard to express how upset you are by pressing down on a little button on a cell phone. To make a very long and drawn-out story short, my paperwork was lost, which caused my disability pay to be delayed.

The chemo was working extra hard on my brain. My journal during this time was full of disjointed sentences. Whereas Tim didn't have any chemotherapy-induced problems, he was feeling the pressure of an empty bank account. On top of everything else he did, he took a few odd jobs to bring in some income. This got him out of the house and allowed him to think about something else. He didn't want to leave me, but I convinced him it was OK. We both knew there were plenty of people who had made themselves available in the event I needed assistance, but Tim still felt guilty about leaving me alone.

Caregivers should be reminded that it's OK to get away from us from time to time. I've read that some caregivers secretly wish they could have free time and then feel guilty for merely having the thought. Mental health professionals say those who are in the support role will be more effective at helping their sick loved one if they care for themselves first. If you've ever traveled on an airplane, you've heard the flight attendant say, "Should the cabin lose pressure, oxygen masks will drop from the overhead area. Please place the mask over your own mouth and nose before assisting others." The same goes for caregivers; if you can't help yourself, how can you help anyone else?

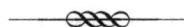

In spite of the warm weather, there were nights when I was cold. The side effects I experienced were all over the map. One thing that was constant was the achiness. It was getting to the point where my poor body hurt to the touch. I didn't want hugs or even pats on the back. This didn't sit well with Tim. He felt alone and wanted companionship. I will not discuss what we went through or how we handled this, as it is very personal, but I will mention a professional's insight on this touchy subject. Stanford Medicine's website on surviving cancer has a section titled "When Your Spouse Has Cancer." This segment explains how cancer (and its treatment) will affect a person's sexual interest and could leave the person feeling depressed and unattractive. It suggests using frank and open communication and recommends that you reassure one another of your commitment.[28]

A friend of ours, whose wife had faced stage-four cancer, encouraged us in this area. He said their relationship had gotten so much stronger since she had been diagnosed. To sum it up, talk

---

[28] "When Your Spouse Has Cancer," Stanford Medicine, http://med.stanford.edu/survivingcancer/cancer-and-stress/when-your-spouse-has-cancer.html.

with each other; speak with your doctors; and don't be afraid to pray about it. "What? Pray about sex?" you ask. Yes, God made sex. If you'd like a good laugh and, at the same time, would like to gain insight into how you can be honest with our heavenly Father about *anything*, look up blogger J. Parker's "A Prayer for Your Sexual Intimacy."[29]

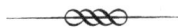

I was tired and hurt all over. I had sores on and in my body and was bald. My teeth ached, my left eye throbbed, I was moody, and food tasted like *yuck*! Sleep evaded me, and I couldn't think straight. With all these signs, you would think that I would have figured out that I was sick, but that was something I didn't want to admit. Let me explain.

One warm night in August, we made the trip to a not-so-nearby city to celebrate Tim's son, Dave's, birthday. I was uncomfortable going out to a crowded eatery and worried about spending money we didn't have. I felt ugly and out of place, even though I tried to spruce up my looks by applying the makeup tricks I had learned from the Look Good, Feel Better class. I just wanted to climb down into a hole and sit there by myself.

The restaurant was packed and noisy. By the sound of it, everyone there was having a grand ol' time. You could hear glasses clinking and entire tables of people laughing at the punch line of a funny joke. It seemed like every person there was smiling and enjoying the evening. When the guest of honor showed up, I didn't recognize him. Dave had gotten a new haircut and was now sporting a mustache. I apologized to him for not realizing who he was right away and laughed that he probably didn't recognize me either, as he

---

[29] J. Parker, "A Prayer for Your Sexual Intimacy," Hot, Holy & Humorous, January 28, 2017, https://hotholyhumorous.com/2017/01/28/a-prayer-for-your-sexual-intimacy.

hadn't seen me in a wig. What he said next touched me deeply: "No, you look beautiful. You look just beautiful."

> Pleasant words are like a honeycomb, Sweetness to the soul and health to the bones. (Proverbs 16:24)

Try it sometime, just a random kind word to someone. It really will refresh their spirit. There was a time when I went to the grocery store and was not totally comfortable with how I looked. My hair had started to grow back, and it was hard to fit the wig on over it, even though it had grown only about an inch and a half long. My spirit was low, and I wasn't feeling 100 percent. As I passed a complete stranger, she looked at me and told me how much she admired my hair. I was so touched by her kind words. I didn't know this woman from Adam, yet she lifted me up just by giving me a little compliment. After I picked up what I needed in that aisle, I sought her out to thank her. As it turned out, her husband was in the throes of his cancer treatment, and they too were low on money. We said we would hold each other up in prayer. I thanked God all the way home for that encounter.

Now, back to the restaurant ...

I felt that the lighting was a bit too low. When the waiter escorted us to our table, I found I wasn't the only one who thought so, as Dave took out his trusty cell phone and used the flashlight app to read the menu. The waiter returned and presented us with a bowl of pickles. Not bread, like most restaurants. No, this restaurant gave us pickles. These were not just any pickles; these were huge, nasty, spicy pickles. *Nothing goes better with a body full of chemo than that.* If I had not been sick, I suppose I would have welcomed the crisp half-sours. As it was, I was starving and decided it was much better to consume this unusual appetizer than chow down on the arm of my chair. I took a small bite, but the pungent pickle packed a punch. On second thought, the chair was starting to look appetizing.

When the food arrived, I was pleasantly surprised to find it tasted very good. Unfortunately, with every morsel I chewed, the flavor soon turned sour, and I finally had to call it a night when I felt like I was pouring salt down my gullet. By the time we left, I was quite frustrated and cried all the way home. It was then that it finally hit me that I was sick. I had been fighting off admitting this for almost five months. Now, reality came crashing down on me like a nine-hundred-pound hailstone. I finally acknowledged to myself that I had cancer.

Chapter 10

I WOULD RATHER DIE OF PASSION THAN OF BOREDOM–VINCENT VAN GOGH

By this time, after much thought and prayer, I decided against removing my healthy breast, so I would *only* be having a unilateral mastectomy. I spoke with Dr. Nett and asked him what I should expect to see after the mastectomy. I didn't want any surprises. He explained that he would perform the first half of the surgery by removing the innards of my breast, including the nipple, areola, and a few sentinel lymph nodes. Doctors nowadays try to spare as much of the breast skin as possible. This makes reconstruction somewhat easier, and it looks more natural. Of course, this all depends on where and how big the masses are.

The nodes he was going to excise, located in the underarm area, carry fluid called lymph through parts of the body to help fight infection and remove toxins. Years ago, when a woman had a mastectomy, many of her nodes would be removed, just in case the cancer had spread. Now, depending upon how advanced the cancer is, only the sentinel nodes—the first few lymph nodes into which a tumor drains—are removed. The medical field found that axillary lymph node removal, which typically involves removal of fifteen to twenty-five nodes, can have serious consequences. When a large amount of the tiny round nodes is removed, lymph fluid might not be able to flow, resulting in lymphedema (a buildup of this fluid). This can cause swelling, as well as problems like limited range of motion, numbness, and pain.[30] The sentinel nodes are biopsied to see if the cancer has spread to the axilla (underarm) lymph nodes. If not, there is no need to remove them all.

Dr. Nòvel would take over for the second half of the surgery. This would be the beginning of my reconstruction. He would insert a temporary skin expander. In my opinion, it was shaped a little odd. This special implant wasn't soft, like a permanent one, and had a tiny valve mechanism that enabled Dr. Nòvel to periodically inject saline to enlarge it. (I was given an implant identification card, as the metal port in the tissue expander might activate airport security devices. In addition, one should avoid having any MRIs done while this expander is in place.) All this to say, after surgery, I would look down and see a nipple-less breast. That lifted a ton off my shoulders. I don't know how I would have reacted to seeing myself with only one breast. Having to face this prospect firsthand gave me compassion toward women who don't or can't have reconstruction.

If anyone in your life has gone through breast cancer, I implore you to not criticize the decisions she made in this regard. This wasn't easy for her. She must look in the mirror and live with her choices. In some cases, it's not even her choice. Between infections and repeated revision surgeries, reconstruction sometimes is just not practical. Thankfully, there are support groups, like Flat & Fabulous, that are "committed to advocating and providing support for those who are living post mastectomy without reconstruction." I saw a study

---

[30] Shari Roan, "Early Stage Breast Cancer: Do You Really Need Your Lymph Nodes Removed?" Everyday Health Group, last updated October 25, 2017, https://www.everydayhealth.com/breast-cancer/treatment/breast-cancer-you-really-need-your-lymph-nodes-removed.

that was published in the journal *JAMA Surgery*[31] that said nearly 59 percent of the women enrolled in the survey chose *not* to have reconstructive surgery. That surprised me. The same study found that regardless of what the women decided, just about 87 percent of them were satisfied with their decision. I think that is a by-product of women being more informed and proactive in their care. They are making decisions they can live with.

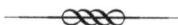

All summer long, I couldn't wait to have surgery. Now that the time was drawing closer and becoming a reality, I was not so eager. I started referring to it in my journal as the "amputation." I imagined the pain I would be in. Then I thought about Habakkuk (*wouldn't anyone?*) Habakkuk was an Old Testament prophet during a very low time in Judah's history. The twelve tribes of Israel had split into two kingdoms—eleven tribes in the north and the tribe of Judah to the south. The northern kingdom had been exiled to Syria. Now, Judah was in danger of being taken over by Babylon and having all its citizens exiled. Those faithful to the Lord, like Habakkuk, were wondering where God was in all of this. The book of Habakkuk is only three chapters long and contains a dialogue between the prophet and God. In it, Habakkuk asks God, "O LORD, how long shall I cry, And You will not hear? Even cry out to You, "Violence!" And You will not save" (Habakkuk 1:2). (You might be thinking these same words—"Where *are* You, God?") He wanted God to *do* something. Eventually, though, Habakkuk's frustration turned into prayers and then praise to God. He stated that even though things go terribly wrong, he would praise and rejoice in God. He

---

[31] M. Morrow, Y. Li, AK Alderman, R. Jagsi, AS Hamilton, JJ Graff, ST Hawley, SJ Katz, "Access to Breast Reconstruction after Mastectomy and Patient Perspectives on Reconstruction Decision Making," *JAMA Surg.* 149, no. 10 (October 2014):1015–21, doi: 10.1001/jamasurg.2014.548. PMID: 25141939; PMCID: PMC4732701. https://www.ncbi.nlm.nih.gov/pmc/articles/PMC4732701.

acknowledged that God is his strength and talked about the blessings he had received from the Almighty.[32]

Bad things happen. Scary things happen. Life is not fair, and we must face unpleasant or even horrifying events. That doesn't mean God is not there. It doesn't mean He has drawn back His hand and won't save. As Habakkuk admitted, God will enable you to endure it. A mountain goat still has to walk on rough, steep, rocky, terrain, but it has the *equipment* to do it.

God will provide what I need when I need it (like manna), and all I need to do is trust in His sovereignty. I wrote a quote by author Bryan Davis in my journal: "Never forget what you learned in the light when you are in the dark." In other words, I know God's character doesn't change. He's taken care of me so far. I have no reason to believe He won't do it now that times are hard. I remembered the verse in Isaiah: "But he was pierced for our transgressions, he was crushed for our iniquities; the punishment that brought us peace was on him, and by his wounds we are healed" (Isaiah 53:4 NIV).

Notice that the verse is written in past tense, but the last statement—"by his wounds we are healed"—is in present tense. I *am* healed; I just have to go through this journey to get there. It's like being paid with a check. When I receive the payment via this form of currency, I don't have the cash in my hand, but I have a signature on the piece of paper that assures me the money is there. Sometimes, I must wait three business days for a check to clear, but I'll get it. I began to think of my healing like that. My healing is assured because the signature on the check is my Savior's blood on the cross. The debt has been paid in full. I realize that not everyone is physically healed of their infirmities, but if they trust Jesus Christ as their Lord and Savior, they have the promise given in Revelation 21:4: "And God will wipe away every tear from their eyes; there shall

---

[32] Habakkuk 3:17–19a.

be no more death, nor sorrow, nor crying. There shall be no more pain, for the former things have passed away."

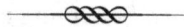

Summer had been lean and painful, but now Labor Day was behind me, and September brought a double blessing. First, we finally received a disability check. And second, Dr. Dawn informed me that today would be my last chemo treatment! The reason it ended a bit earlier than expected all started with sand in my shoes. At least, I thought it was sand. Every day, a few times a day, I would take off my socks and shoes, empty out my shoes (there was never anything in them, other than my feet), and rub the bottoms of my toes to clear it of the debris I thought was there. It was a very strange sensation. As Dr. Dawn examined me, she nonchalantly asked, "So how's your neuropathy?"

My mouth dropped open, and the light bulb went on! "So *that's* what that is!" I exclaimed. I knew a little bit about this disease because my mother had suffered from it. Neuropathy happens when there is nerve damage. It can cause tingling, numbness, and other sensations (like feeling sand between your toes), often in the feet and hands. Dr. Dawn ended the chemo because she didn't want the neuropathy to get worse. Evidently, neuropathy may reverse itself and stop after the chemo treatments end. As of this writing, I still have a little sand left in my socks, but it's not as bad as it was.

Ending chemo gave me a huge morale boost. I wanted to keep that positive attitude, so for me, I absolutely had to stay *off* social media. The negativity was beginning to get to me. The only time I ventured out into the virtual world was to post a "*What?!*" Fact of the Day on Facebook. My definition of this is as follows: random, lack of pattern or predictability, not crucial, unexpected, as in out of the blue. It is a random fact that intentionally leaves out the minutiae. I hope that doing this will pique readers' interest so they'll dig more deeply into the topic, which will expand their knowledge of useless information. For instance: "Many cereals are fortified with added iron. These cereals, when crushed to a powdery consistency, can be picked up using a strong magnet." *What?!* See what I mean? Don't you just want to find out more about that?

Going to church every week also helped to keep me sane and grounded. One of the songs we sing is by the group Vertical Worship, called "Yes, I Will." The lyrics to this song really resonated with me; here are a few that I wrote in my journal.

> I count on one thing
> The same God that never fails
> Will not fail me now
> You won't fail me now
> In the waiting
> The same God who's never late
> Is working all things out
> You're working all things out

Since chemo was over, Drs. Nett and Nòvel were waiting for my strength to return before they performed surgery. They say that chemo is out of your body quickly, but the effects linger.[33] Dr. Dawn always encouraged me to drink a lot of water while I was being infused, but she never mentioned any actions I should take after completing my treatment. Some doctors will advise their patients to detoxify after chemo; others do not think it beneficial. After discussing it with Dr. Dawn, I decided to drink detox tea and take hot Epsom salt baths. Epsom salt, made from both magnesium and sulfate, is not the same as table salt, which is made from sodium. The minerals in Epsom salt draw out toxins from the body and soothe sore, achy muscles. I had already incorporated many of the foods suggested to aid in this process, but I added cranberries and fatty

---

[33] "How Chemotherapy Affects Your Body after Treatment," WebMD.com, June 7, 2020, https://www.webmd.com/cancer/post-chemo-body-changes#1.

fish, like tuna. The term *fatty fish* sounds unappealing, but these fish are the healthiest to consume. They are chock-full of omega-3 fatty acids. These are *good* fats. (Who knew there was such a thing?)

By September 14, only two weeks since my last chemo treatment, I noticed that I had peach fuzz on my head. My hair was growing back! I was so excited. Add to that a phone call from Dr. Nett, who advised me that my surgery was scheduled and was less than a month away.

I'd been waiting for this day for months, and now that I knew exactly when it was, fear clenched me with a death grip. Not a rational, logical dread that one might have when facing the loss of a body part. No, I was overwhelmed with the paralyzing thought that I would have to be in an enclosed death trap—*an elevator*! I know it sounds trivial, but I have come to know, on a very intimate level, that phobias are excessive and irrational. I would have to take one or two for this surgery, and the mere thought horrified me.

I tried to focus on the good things, like how my body was starting to heal. I could tell I was recovering because food began to taste better, and the sores on my arms and face were fading. Although I tired easily, I ventured out of the house by myself, and it felt great! I also prepared for surgery by purchasing items I needed post-op. Dr. Nòvel suggested I get two compression bras and a comfortable outfit to wear home after surgery. The latter was easy to find. I bought soft cotton sweatpants and a zippered hoodie. The bras, however, were difficult to locate. I tried the mall, but none of the undergarments there fit the bill. I had to order them online from a company that specialized in medical-grade compression garments. The bras (even with a discount code) were nearly ninety dollars each. That might not sound like much to some, but to me, each bra was almost two weeks' worth of groceries.

Dr. Nòvel gave me prescriptions for pain meds (no Percocet), an antibiotic to ward off any infections, and one scopolamine patch. The transdermal patch is the same one you get if you're going on a cruise and are susceptible to seasickness. It helps fight nausea.

Autumn was here, and the days were getting cooler. We attended

Harvest Fest, an event our church hosts annually, as a last hurrah before surgery. It was nice to enjoy the seasonal foods (sweet potato and apple pies, cider, and anything pumpkin-flavored); the last of the warm sunshine; bands that performed harmonic ballads, contemporary Christian, and doo-wop music; pumpkin painting; a petting zoo; a clown who twisted balloons into shapes, from swords and crowns to poodles; face painting; and cheeseburgers, hot dogs, and Grace's famous french fries.

The fries were made from the largest spuds I'd ever seen. You'd only need two to make a scalloped potato casserole. We've been known to go through nearly eight hundred of the tubers. There was a team of volunteers who used a machine to cut up the potatoes and then cook 'em up in one of the many propane-powered deep fryers.

There were oodles of squealing children impatiently waiting in lines to jump around in the various bounce houses. I joined the line to grab a homemade empanada with spicy salsa, and it was *delicioso*! This distraction was much needed and appreciated.

The Sunday before surgery, the elders of our church gathered before the service to anoint me with oil, lay hands on me, and pray. They asked detailed questions so the prayers would be specific. Foster was there, so I felt comfortable confiding in him about my apprehension of being enclosed in an elevator. Much to my surprise, no one laughed or made me feel like my request was silly. On the contrary, they took it seriously. One of our dear friends (we call her Prayin' Pat) asked God to free me from this phobia and make it the polar opposite, where I wouldn't even think about traveling in elevators and eventually would take them just for the fun of it. I had never thought of elevators and fun in the same context, but I liked that request. She also told me to pray against any fear that tried to subdue me, even speaking it out loud, if need be. *Yeshua* is Hebrew for Jesus. This wonderful name means "to rescue, to save, or to deliver."

> The LORD is my rock and my fortress and my deliverer. (2 Samuel 22:2b)

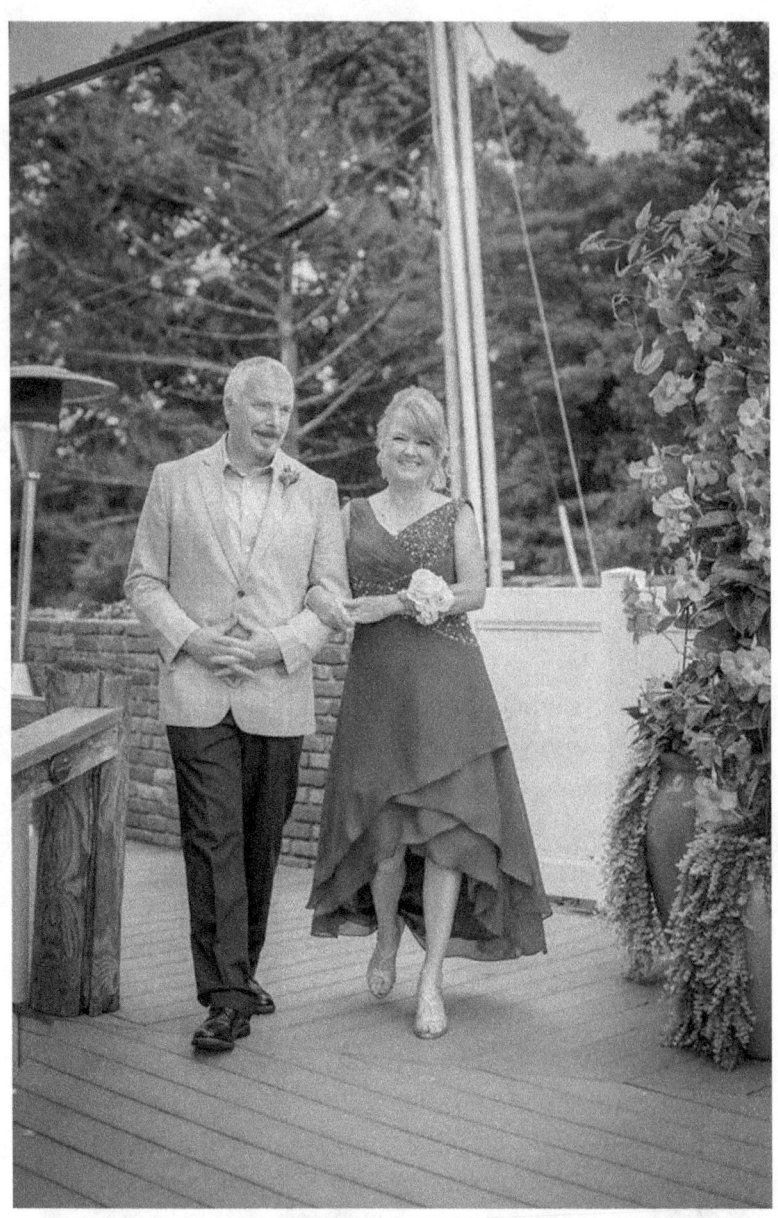

Tim and me, celebrating Erin and Kevin's wedding "down the shore." This was just about eight months before I received the dreaded diagnosis.

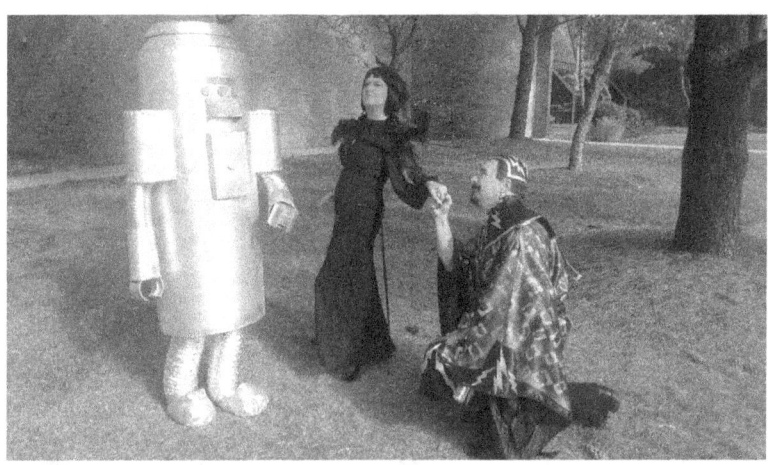

Rosa, me, and Tim, portraying characters from the starship *Voyager*'s hologram program, *Captain Proton,* at a *Star Trek* convention.

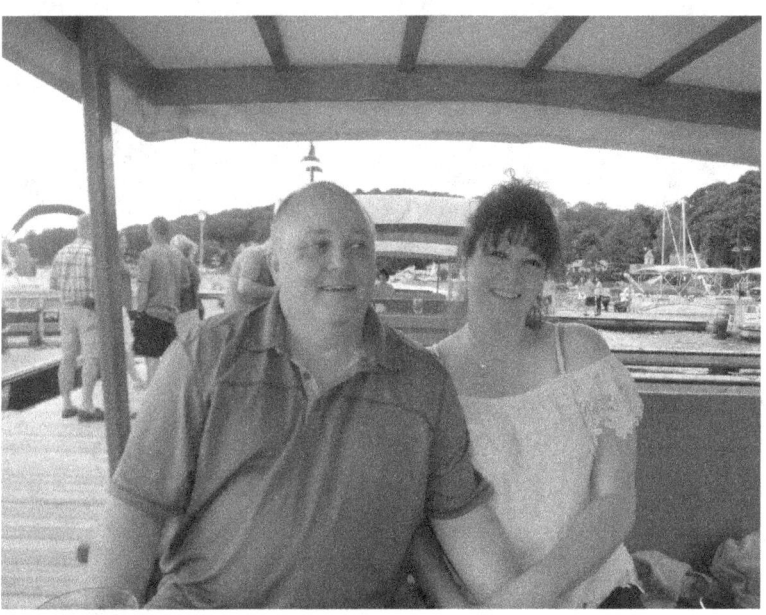

Rosa and Keir on one of their many happy adventures.

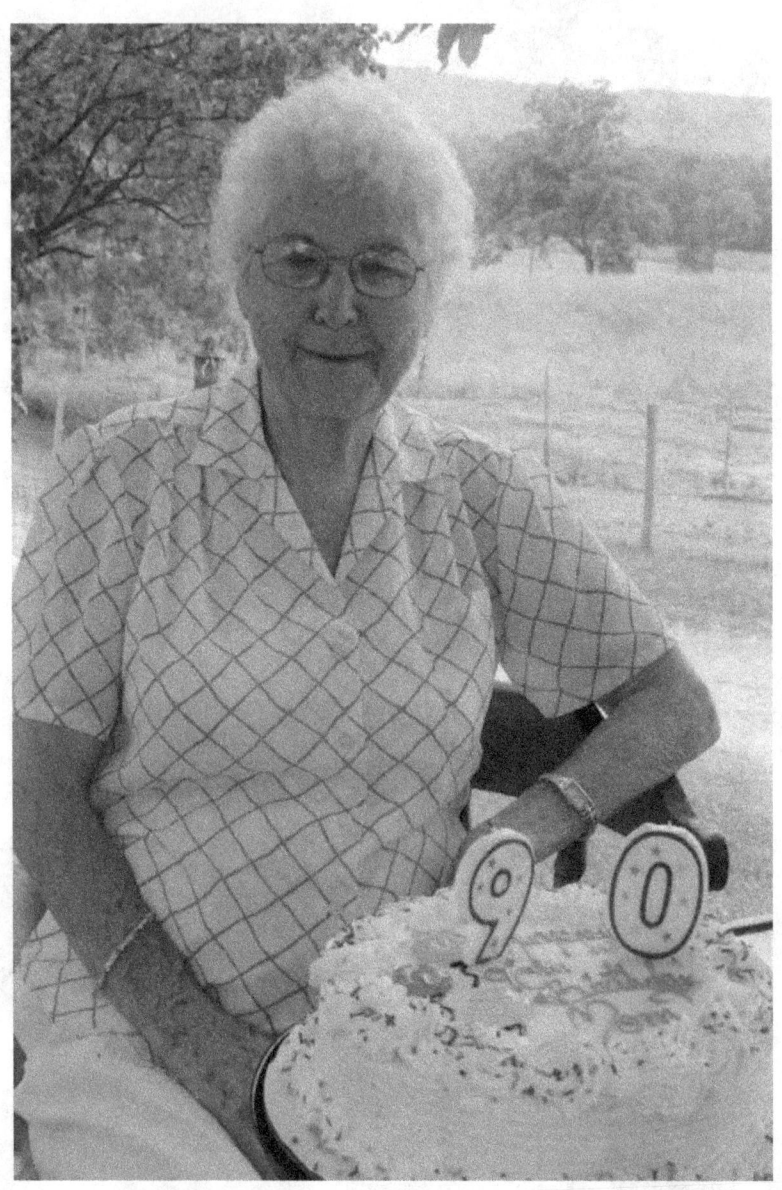

Mom, celebrating her ninetieth trip around the sun.

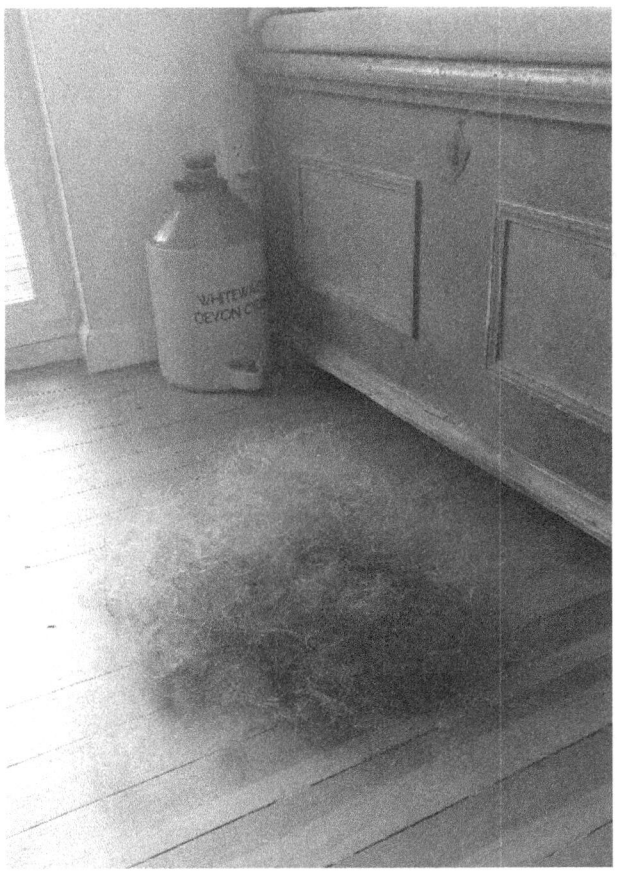

This was the massive pile of hair that fell out in one sitting!
Believe it or not, I still had some left on my head.

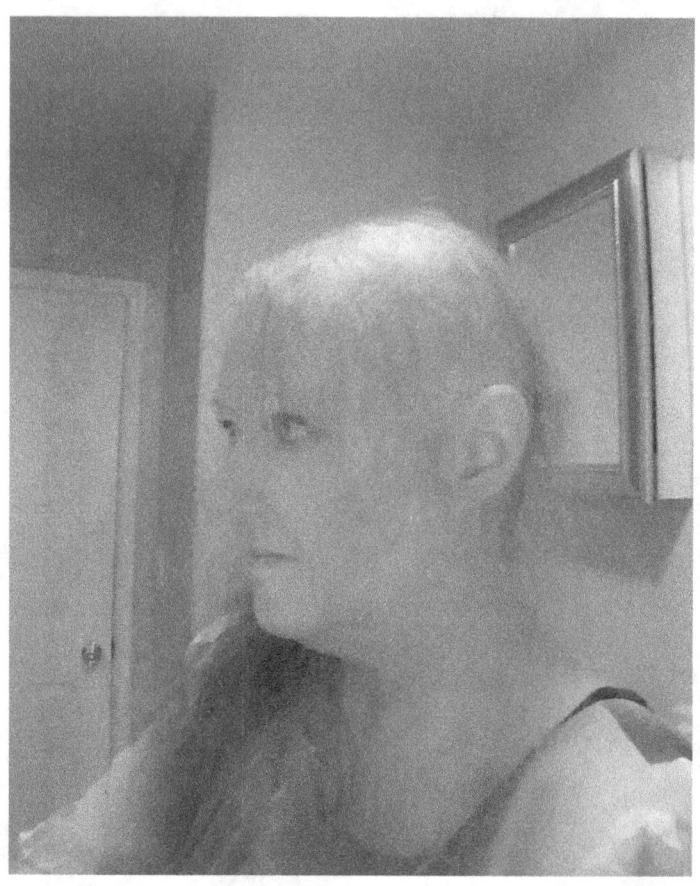

When my hair felt the effects of the chemo, I began, in my mind, to quite closely resemble the Toxic Avenger.

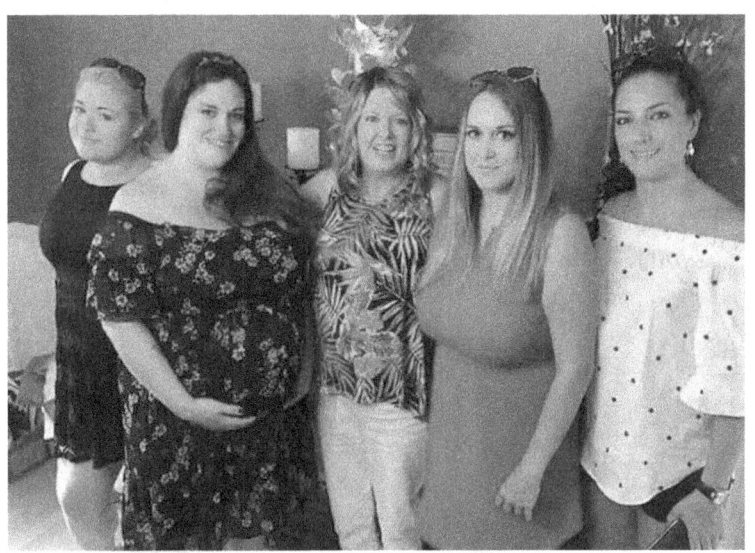

My baby girl Juliet; mommy-to-be Erin; me, with my hair prosthesis; middle sister, Alyson; and Tim's daughter Rebecca, all enjoying our day at River's baby shower.

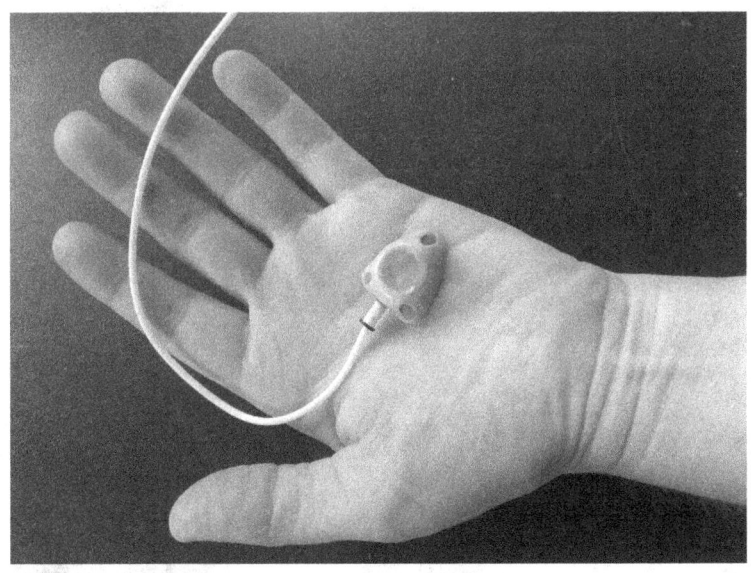

This tiny port—or as I refer to it, Borg implant—was once in my chest. Some women turn their ports into decorative necklaces to remind themselves how far they have come.

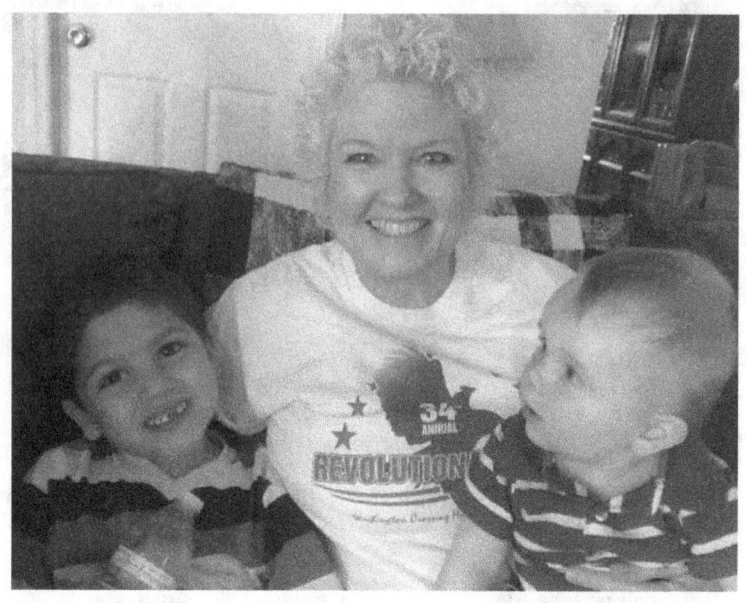
Nina, glowing with pride, with her two boys, Blaise (left) and River (right).

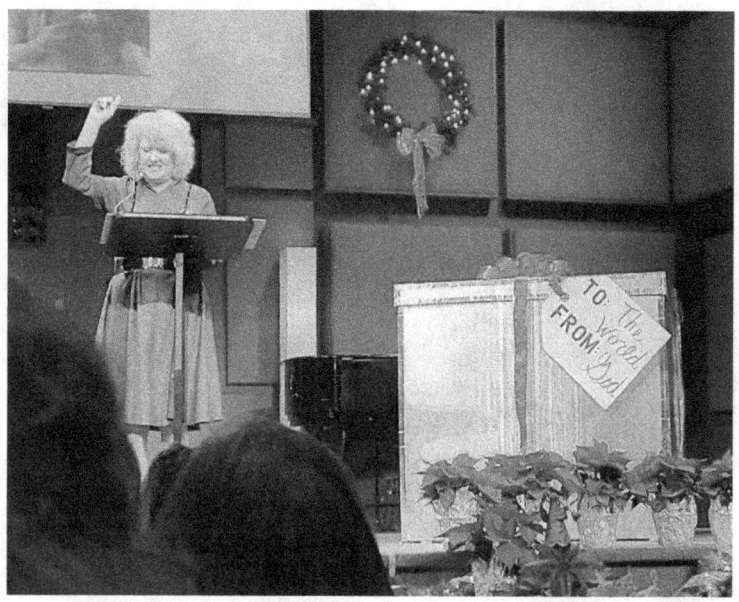
Despite my wild hair and a dress that didn't fit, speaking to my newfound friends about the greatest gift ever was exhilarating!

Chapter 11

EVERY STRIKE BRINGS ME CLOSER TO THE NEXT HOME RUN—BABE RUTH

T-minus one day! On Sunday night, my instructions were to shower using a special antiseptic/antimicrobial skin cleanser called Hibiclens that killed germs for twenty-four hours after it was used. I was to wash normally and then cover my body, from my neck down, with it; turn off the water; and let it sit on my skin for five minutes before rinsing it off. Brrr! I also was told to sleep in freshly washed pajamas and sheets that night.

The next day found me refreshed and in a wonderful mood. The Bible verse in my devotional was very encouraging and one that kept popping up all throughout this journey: "The LORD your God in your midst, The Mighty One, will save; He will rejoice over you with gladness, He will quiet you with His love, He will rejoice over you with singing" (Zephaniah 3:17).

I have to admit that I had peace, but I was not looking forward to the day's events. And even though I had washed last night, I was instructed to take another shower that morning, using just the special cleanser.

We arrived at the hospital and went up to the surgical floor. (I took the stairs.) I was presented with a hospital gown, cap, and socks. I hated that I couldn't wear contact lenses, make-up, or my wig. I looked about one hundred years old! I was then told that I had to have a scan. This scan, called a *lymphoscintigraph*, would enable Dr. Nett to determine which nodes would be removed. First, I had to have a radioactive substance, called a tracer, and blue dye injected into my breast. They warned me that this might sting. What they should have warned me about was the miniscule size of the machine that I would be squished into!

A very pleasant orderly came, and off the three of us went, bed and all. We had to go down to the radiology department. I shut my eyes as tightly as I could. I knew the bed was big and the elevator was small, and I did *not* want to see it. I felt the bump of the wheels as they went over the elevator door's track. I heard the *bing* as the doors slowly closed. Before I felt the slight jerk as the elevator started its descent, I heard Tim's phone blasting Charles Jenkins's gospel hit, "This Means War"! With trombones blaring and syncopated tambourines and clapping, the elevator was filled with the comforting lyrics:

> I got joy in my soul
> God is in control
> I got Satan on my trail
> But I'm singing all is well
> He's attacking everyday
> But I'm watching while I pray
> No matter the attack
> I won't turn back

Still with my eyes tightly closed, I felt the elevator stop, and I thought we had arrived, but no! People on another floor had pushed the call button, and we made an unscheduled stop. Tim told me later that when the doors opened, the prospective riders realized there was no room for them and stepped back to wait, but as they did, they began to sway and nod their heads to the moving gospel rhythm that emanated from the car. As all this was going on, I was concentrating with all my heart on a sermon I had heard recently. The pastor had talked about God's Shekinah glory. Shekinah is from the Hebrew word *shākan*, which means "to reside or permanently stay." This is a visible manifestation of God on earth, whose presence is portrayed through a natural occurrence, sometimes like a cloud. I pictured this and marveled at how safe I felt when I was near God's presence.

We finally arrived on the correct floor, and when the doors opened, I inhaled deeply, but I didn't open my eyes until I felt the wheels of my bed bump-bump over the door track. Tim had to wait outside, with my bed, while I was brought into a small room with monitors, computers, and (in my opinion) a teeny-tiny MRI-like machine. The nurses assisted me onto a hard, flat surface, which, much to my chagrin, would pull me inside this miniscule scanner. I wanted to run out of the room. I felt like crying. Instead, I concentrated on breathing steadily and regularly. I thought about how important this procedure was and that my God would be with me and get me through this ordeal. I didn't want to verbalize it, but I confessed to the nurse that I was claustrophobic. She could see I was afraid and explained that there were three parts to this scan where I would be inside the machine. To ease my discomfort, she would take me out after each one.

It really did hurt when the tracer was injected into the soft part of my underarm, but I didn't care. The pain of being stuffed into this contraption was far greater than any injection. Unlike the MRI that I'd had back in April, this machine was so tight that when I was slowly drawn in, my nose nearly touched the inside of the scanner. My heart was racing. I had to turn my head to the side so I wouldn't feel the warmth of my breath and hear the echo of it as I exhaled. I was lying on my side, with one arm up over my head and the other arm kind of twisted, so my hand stuck out the opposite side. A counselor came into the room and held my hand to calm me, but it didn't work. I remembered how I was comforted by concentrating on God's Shekinah glory. I knew Jesus was with me. I thought about how Jesus was with Meshach, Shadrach, and Abednego in the fiery furnace. I didn't care how small this space was; there was enough room for Him in here too!

That part of the scan was over, and the platform slowly moved me out of the machine's embrace. I took a deep breath and savored the open air. Much too soon, I was on my way back in. This time, I knew what to expect and was terrified. The counselor had left the room so there was no one there to hold my hand. How I wished Tim could be there. I turned my head again, and the picture of a wide-open field entered my mind. With it came the sensation of a cool breeze wafting over the grass. I truly felt like I was in a wide-open space.

Once again, I was brought out. The nurse was busy typing something into the computer that controlled this tiny monster. *Last one*, I thought as I was pulled back inside for the final scan. Again, I was transported to the beautiful green field. I was so grateful and felt calmer. I was humbled by God's deliverance.

When the scans were completed a nurse helped me up and I stumbled out into the hallway and back onto my bed. The orderly pushed me down the hall to the elevator. And once again Charles Jenkins sang his heart out:

> I plead the blood, I plead, I plead the blood
> There's power in the blood (I plead, I plead the blood)
> Healing in the blood …

With my eyes squeezed shut, I grabbed hold of what I thought was Tim's hand, but I had latched on to the orderly's hand. I don't think that sweet man had ever experienced the likes of me! When the doors opened, I was so relieved. In my mind, what had just happened was the *hard part*.

As we rounded the corner and got back to my room, I found

a wonderful double-surprise waiting for me. Erin and Alyson were there to wish me well and comfort me. Indeed, they did! I realized it wasn't easy for either of them to make the trip. Not that the hospital was extremely far away, but Erin's due date was in twenty-four hours, and I knew she was uncomfortable. (She wore a maternity top with a picture of a popsicle on it that read, "Ready to Pop!") I was also aware that Alyson had to make concessions with work to rearrange her schedule to be here. I appreciated both their efforts. Then they put the cherry on top and called Juliet and Blaise to have a FaceTime chat. I felt so blessed. There's nothing in the world like knowing your kids love you.

A nurse came in and interrupted all the chatter to tell me I had to disinfect—as if all the washing I had already done wasn't enough. I was instructed on how to systematically wash myself down with six special, large, sopping-wet antiseptic wipes. I also had to brush my teeth and tongue with mouthwash and swab out my nose with orange antibacterial goo. All this cleaning was to prevent the possibility of infection. They were taking no chances, and that was all right with me. The only thing left now was to hurry up and wait.

Soon enough, the nurse came in and told me it was showtime. I said my goodbyes and assured everyone I would be OK. Since I had to leave my glasses with Tim, I couldn't see much. The anesthesiologist came over to talk to me and asked me about my patch. Next, Dr. Nett and Dr. Nòvel stood over me, and I told them I had been praying for them. I was surprised when Dr. Nett responded, "There's no need. You'll be OK." I'm not sure what he meant by that. I suppose he sees many people who pray only when they are frightened, and he did not want that for me, but I was not afraid.

If you've ever been in an OR, you know two things: they're cold, and they're usually not very large. I thought I would need a bigger operating room because there was a whole procession going into the room. I'm not talking about all the doctors, nurses, technicians, and orderlies. My procession was as follows: first, Jesus went before me.

Then, as I went in, I was surrounded by a host of strong, tall, fiery, fierce angels,* carrying large swords. Then, Jesus went behind me. Finally, there were my prayer warriors. I don't know how many of them went in, but I pictured at least one hundred. I thought about how Dr. Nett would react if he could see my entourage, and I chuckled to myself.

I wanted to get this over with. The surgery took about four and a half hours. Unbeknownst to me, Rosa showed up at the hospital to sit with Tim. When my surgery was done and I was in recovery, she came in to see me and started crying. She said I looked like I was dead. *Well, of course!* I wasn't wearing any makeup or wig, and I was so cold that my skin was as pale as the sheets on the bed. She had never seen me without all my beauty enhancements. It's amazing what a little greasepaint will do. I always laugh when guys say they like women who sport a natural appearance. You know what I mean. These men have no idea how much primping and makeup go into giving women that look!

The next thing I remember, I was being put into a bed by a gaggle of nurses. I opened my eyes, said "I feel sick," and promptly threw up. After that, I felt great—tired but fine. My Tim came in to see me, and he looked like something the cat dragged in. I could tell he was worried and very tired. I'm not sure he had eaten anything all day. I told him I was fine and that he should go home and get some rest. Unfortunately, my glasses went with him.

I didn't sleep very soundly, but that was to be expected in the hospital. My blood pressure was taken every hour or so, and I had IPC (intermittent pneumatic compression) cuffs on my legs (although only one was working). These cuffs were wrapped around my calves, and every so often, they filled with air and squeezed my legs. This was to increase blood flow and help prevent blood clots.

Note: I would need to write another book to go into detail about angels, but according to the Bible: (1) we don't become angels when we die. That's a fable from the classic Christmas movie It's a Wonderful Life; *and (2) angels in the Bible are not depicted like the cute blond sweethearts we see on Hallmark Christmas cards.*

Every time it filled with air, I woke up. And I don't care how quiet the hospital staff tried to be; I couldn't help but hear the myriad pages over the speakers during the night. In the words of Samuel Goldwyn, "A hospital is no place to be sick."

In the morning, Dr. Nòvel came in to check on me. I was groggy, and, of course, I couldn't see him. He examined my breast and said he was happy with the looks of everything; he emptied both drains. He told me the nurse would show me how to do this, and he'd see me in about two weeks. I was well enough to go home.

Drains are long tubes that are inserted into the breast area and armpit to collect excess fluid. There are plastic bulbs at the end of the tubes that create suction, which keeps the blood and lymphatic fluid from collecting under the skin. It's held in place with a stitch or two.

When Tim came to pick me up, it took both him and the nurse to get me dressed. It was then that I realized the compression brassieres were worth every penny. I'd never seen so many hook-and-eye clasps on a bra before. There were three rows of eight on the front closure and then three rows of four on each shoulder. It was more like a vest. When you have drains, bandages, and stitches, all these openings are invaluable. The grenade part of the drains was safety pinned to my bra so it didn't get yanked out (*ouch*!) or dangle beneath my shirt. (Wouldn't *that* have looked attractive!)

Maria, my visiting nurse, came to see me at home two to three times to measure pain levels, take my temperature, inspect the wounds, and document drainage. She showed me the Wong–Baker pain scale. That's the technical name for those pictures of the little faces to help you best describes your "ouch." I kept telling her it was only a four, but Maria could tell I wasn't being very forthcoming. She could see my eyes were watering from the discomfort. She knew I was reticent to take anything for the pain. We finally figured out that if I took acetaminophen with a Valium, the pain was manageable.

Sleeping was not comfortable for a few weeks. I couldn't lie on my back and most definitely not on my side. I had to sleep propped up with pillows. If I needed to use the facilities during the night, I had to wake Tim, as I could not use my left arm to leverage myself out of the bed. I cannot imagine how difficult all this must be for women who have had a double mastectomy.

During this recovery time, I read a devotional and received a wonderful, comforting verse from God. Remember how I said I felt like I was in a wide-open field when I was crammed into the lymphoscintigraph scanner? Check out this verse: "He brought me out into a spacious place; he rescued me because he delighted in me" (Psalm 18:19 NIV). Although physically I'd been imprisoned inside a body-hugging scanner, He truly brought me out into a spacious place, complete with a breeze!

I read up on what that could have meant to King David, who wrote this psalm. Even though David had been anointed king over Israel by the prophet Samuel when he was young (maybe a late teen), he didn't get to physically reign until he was thirty years old. During those years, David served the reigning monarch, Saul, who was jealous of David. There are many instances where Saul tried to kill David. As a result, David found himself fleeing from Saul's wrath and hiding in caves. For David, to be in a wide-open space meant a state of freedom; not surrounded by traps, or enemies waiting in ambush. Yes, God had surely given me great comfort in a place of safety.

Ten days after surgery, I was scheduled to see Dr. Nòvel. I was hoping he'd take the drains out, as they were uncomfortable. Plus, it was hard to find clothing that concealed them, unless I wore a muumuu.

I wasn't the only one who was uncomfortable. Erin had gone well over a week past her due date and was enormously ready to deliver. Every time the phone rang, we were sure it was going to be the news that River had come into the world, but we heard nothing.

It was slow going, but I made it to Dr. Nòvel's office. While we were waiting in the exam room, I got *the* call! I was so excited and glad that River had waited until I was able to go see him in person. What an accommodating little guy! Even though I was beat up, I wanted to make the trip over to the hospital to see my grandbaby, daughter, and son-in-law. Tim was working odd jobs, so he was unable to go in with me, but he promised he'd be back to peek in on the tired and happy little family as he dropped me off at the hospital. By the way, Dr. Nòvel said my pathology was good and that Dr. Nett would discuss it with me further, but the drains remained in.

The hospital that ushered in my grandson was quite large, with just about seven hundred beds on a forty-acre campus. Of course, where I was and where I had to go were on opposite ends of the building. I was wishing I had a Segway, as I was moving as slow as a turtle. Thankfully, I arrived just in time to see the nurse take River's footprints. He was absolutely beautiful, and Erin, although exhausted from many, many hours of labor, was radiant. I used any strength I had that day to see the newest edition of our family, but it was well worth it.

After a good night's sleep, I was off to see Dr. Nett. I was so sore and tired that I didn't have much time to digest the previous day's events, although my mind was laser-focused on the possibility that I might have to endure radiation treatments, a cancer treatment that uses high doses of radiation to kill cancer cells and shrink tumors. The National Cancer Institute says it does this by damaging cancer's DNA. There are different types of radiation therapy, but the one I was probably looking at was external radiation. During this type of radiation, the high-energy beams come from a machine outside of the body that aims the beams at a precise point on the body. One typically receives this type of radiology treatment on an outpatient basis, five days a week over a certain period. These sessions may last ten to thirty minutes. Of course, there are different treatments, depending on the type of cancer and how advanced it is. Either way, I didn't want it. I had heard it was painful and that skin around the treated area can be red, like a sunburn, and peel. It's also possible to have permanent damage from the radiation, so I wanted to avoid it, if I could.

Dr. Nett and his assistant were happy to see me. He told me my pathology was the best news I could possibly get. He said when he opened me up, he saw no cancer, just scar tissue! In addition, he explained it was usual to see a few cancer cells in the biopsy of excised lymph nodes, but in my case, there was none! His bubbly assistant laughed, jumped up and down, and clapped her hands together at the great news. Dr. Nett, who usually showed little emotion, was grinning ear to ear. I, however, sat there like a bump on a log. I felt ungrateful and rather rude for not showing more enthusiasm. I thought about it all the way home, and then it hit me. I didn't get overly excited or show an outward expression of relief because that was the diagnosis I had expected all along. I knew, in my heart of hearts, that I was going to be OK. I had the assurance that I would be healed by the Great Physician.[34] I shared this experience with Foster at church one Sunday, and he laughed and said he did exactly the same thing! He knew God had rid his body of the cancer. I think we both had the same thought: "This was the LORD's doing; It is marvelous in our eyes" (Psalm 118:23).

---

[34] Bless the Lord, O my soul,
And forget not all His benefits:
Who forgives all your iniquities,
Who heals all your diseases.
(Psalm 103:2–3)

Chapter 12

THE DRAINS GO IN, THE DRAINS COME OUT

Louisa sent me a text to tell me she was getting her port implanted. I was happy, knowing she was getting the help she needed, but I was also sad because I knew firsthand just how awful chemo treatments can be. At about this same time, I heard from another friend, June, to whom I hadn't spoken in years. I sent her an email early on to let her know I had breast cancer. Being a member of Team C, I knew she would understand. June had suffered from breast cancer years ago and had a mastectomy back in the day when all the lymph nodes were removed. She had opted not to have reconstruction. I'll never forget the day she showed me her battle scars. She had just returned home from the hospital, and I had been helping her out by watching her children. She asked me if I wanted to see what had been done. I told her no, but I guess it was a rhetorical question. Nausea welled up inside me when I saw the more than one hundred stitches and staples that laced the area where her breast had been. I think her doctors were more interested in saving her life and not too concerned with aesthetics. I didn't want her to see how upset I was so I excused myself. I quickly went into the powder room and cried.

A few years later, after the tragic death of her toddler son, she moved out of state, and we lost touch with each other. But thanks to social media, we were able to hook up again, and it was great hearing from her. One day, June surprised me with a video call, and I was shocked to see how her health had deteriorated. Her skin was ashen, and she was wearing a nasal cannula (the tube with prongs that fit inside your nose). I couldn't see it, but I heard what I assumed was her portable oxygen machine. Since we had last spoken, June had had a recurrence of breast cancer and had to undergo yet another mastectomy. For a second time, she decided against having reconstruction. She also suffered from COPD (chronic obstructive pulmonary disease). This illness is a lingering inflammatory lung disease that impedes airflow from the lungs. Some of the symptoms include difficulty breathing, cough, mucus production, and wheezing. In June's case, her COPD was caused by a lifetime of cigarette smoking. This was a vice that had haunted her for decades. She always felt defeated because of this, like she wasn't good enough for God. Going to church was next to impossible due to her fragile condition and her oxygen tank, and this saddened her. What she said next, in between gasping for every breath, deeply pierced my very being: "Do you think God is mad at me?"

For whatever reason, she couldn't grasp that God loved her just as she was. Her words broke my heart because it sounded as if she was desperately reaching out for any hope or reassurance that God hadn't turned His back on her. I thought about how hopeless I had felt many years ago, when I tried to please God to somehow win His favor. I wanted to encourage her, to let her know she was loved more than she would ever know.

"My God is gracious, forgiving, and patient," I said in a soft, whisper-like timbre. "My salvation isn't about what I can do for Him but what *He did for me.*"

That was the last time I spoke with my dear friend, as she succumbed to the COPD and went home to be with the Lord a few months later. I thought, *Now, my sweet sister, now you know how much your heavenly Father loves you. Rest in Him, my friend.*[35]

Once more, I sat in convalescent limbo. There wasn't much to do, except soul search while waiting for my body to heal. A timely devotional I read during this period resonated in my heart. In it, the writer explained that she felt unworthiness and shame over her "less-than-godly past." *That was me*, I thought. How could I possibly do God's work with the messed-up life I've lived? Her point was that God accepts us as we are and changes us as we serve Him in love. I once heard someone say, "A dog doesn't bark to become a dog. He barks because he *is* a dog."

If anyone should have lamented over his past life, it was the apostle Paul. When we first read about him in the Bible, he is referred to as Saul, but Saul's name was also Paul. It was common in those days to have dual names. Acts 13:9 describes the apostle as "Saul, who also is called Paul." In scripture, from that verse on, Saul is always referred to as "Paul." He had all the right breeding (born of Jewish parents, a Pharisee from the tribe of Benjamin), powerful citizenship (a Roman), and a respected education (studied the Hebrew scriptures in the city of Jerusalem under the tutelage of Rabbi Gamaliel[36]). Only a few years had passed since the crucifixion and Resurrection of Jesus, and Saul, a self-righteous, religious zealot, was going from house to house, dragging men and women off to prison for their belief in Jesus of Nazareth. Saul was present when Stephen, the first Christian martyr, was stoned to death. He even admitted later that he was in full approval[37] of Stephen's murder. However, Saul of Tarsus was about to have a divine detour on the

---

[35] Read Psalm 130, and see how loving, patient, caring, and forgiving our God is.
[36] Gamaliel was a first-century Jewish rabbi and a leader in the Jewish Sanhedrin. He is mentioned in Acts 5:34 as a famous and well-respected teacher.
[37] Acts 22:20.

road to Damascus, where he was going to continue his brutal pursuit of the church. He came face-to-face, so to speak, with the very One he was persecuting.

> Then Saul, still breathing threats and murder against the disciples of the Lord, went to the high priest and asked letters from him to the synagogues of Damascus, so that if he found any who were of the Way, whether men or women, he might bring them bound to Jerusalem.
>
> As he journeyed he came near Damascus, and suddenly a light shone around him from heaven. Then he fell to the ground, and heard a voice saying to him, "Saul, Saul, why are you persecuting Me?" (Acts 9:1–4)

So in his new life as a believer in Yeshua Hamashiach (Jesus the Anointed One), he had much shame to bear. He carried the pain in his heart that he was the reason so many of the Way (what Christians were called at that time) were imprisoned or dead. How many children had he left without parents? How many widows? How many had to flee their homes and leave all they had? Saul considered himself the biggest sinner of all. "This is a faithful saying and worthy of all acceptance, that Christ Jesus came into the world to save sinners, of whom I am chief" (1 Timothy 1:15). Yet he didn't let this stand in the way of his service to God. Neither should we. "And I thank Christ Jesus our Lord who has enabled me, because He counted me faithful, putting me into the ministry" (1 Timothy 1:12). Yes, I make mistakes, but God's grace is greater than my sin. People are observant. They notice how we act and react to situations to see how this Jesus makes a difference in our lives.

I found one person who was watching: my sweet grandson Blaise. He knew that what was happening to me was bad and scary, but he saw that I wasn't afraid. One day, I received a phone call from Juliet. Blaise was at the doctor's office and had to get a shot. He was terrified, so he asked his mommy if she could please call Nina because he wanted some of Nina's bravery. In the words of the great hymn writer Harry Dixon Loes, "This little light of mine, I'm going to let it shine"!

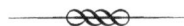

At the instruction of Dr. Nett, I began doing stretching exercises. I was to stand with my shoulder facing the wall with my arm in a sideways, Supremes-type "Stop in the Name of Love" stance. Then, as I slowly moved toward the wall, my arm would rise. I was to do this as far as I could and hold it there for a few seconds. This stretched out the area where the nodes were removed. Dr. Nett said I wouldn't be left with any perennial limitations. I was happy to hear that because I knew people who did have permanent weakness in their arms from the lymphadenectomy. I also realized I had to get better because it wouldn't be long before I had to return to work. It's not like I sat at a desk all day, and I was concerned that I wouldn't have the fortitude to endure all the strenuous work expected of me.

I worried unnecessarily about how I would deal with work and radiation treatments simultaneously. My appointment with the radiation oncologist was short and sweet. She didn't think I needed radiation treatments. That was it. I was thrilled! Now *all* I had to concentrate on was getting well and building my stamina. I was ready to get back to the business of being me again. I didn't know, however, that there was more medicine and chemo headed in my direction. I'll get to that part soon enough.

In the meantime, I received a text message from someone I had not heard from in many years. We got to talking (as it were), and since we had mutual friends, I asked her if she had heard that I had cancer. She responded that she had and that she was praying for me. She then added, "Prayer is powerful."

That statement struck me as odd, and I'll tell you why. I know God is powerful, and He does powerful things through prayer. But I'm not so sure that *prayer*, in and of itself, is powerful. Let me explain. Naturalists believe there are no objectively existing deities. They view the conscious and deliberate exercise of conversing with an imaginary being as having psychological value, kind of like personalizing a journal or speaking out loud to a deceased loved one. According to the Spiritual Naturalist Society, "An imaginary god will do just as well as a real one as any 'answers' to prayer come ultimately from oneself anyway." I ask you to consider if a prayer of that kind is powerful. I think not, as it is to whom one prays that makes the difference.

There's a perfect illustration of this in 1 Kings about a prophet of God named Elijah. Israel had a wicked king by the name of Ahab (you may have heard of his wife, Jezebel). God had had enough of the idolatry of His people and sent Elijah to confront him. Ahab had forsaken God's commandments and worshiped the Baals. (These are false gods.) God was going to have a showdown! Instead of meeting at high noon at the OK Corral, Elijah told Ahab to call all the Israelites, the 450 prophets of Baal, and the 400 prophets of Asherah (another false god) and meet him at Mount Carmel.

> And Elijah came to all the people, and said, "How long will you falter between two opinions? If the LORD is God, follow Him; but if Baal, follow him." But the people answered him not a word. (1 Kings 18:21)

There were crickets. None of the people spoke up. That was it! The time for talking was over! Elijah instructed the prophets to get a bull, prepare it as a sacrifice, and set it up on an altar. Elijah would do the same. Then, neither party would light the fire to burn the sacrifice; instead, the prophets would call on their gods, and Elijah would call on the Lord.

Then you call on the name of your gods, and I will call on the name of the LORD; and the God who answers by fire, He is God" (1 Kings 18:24a)

Everyone agreed this was a good idea. So the pagan prophets took the prepared sacrifice and prayed to Baal from morning until noon but to no avail. These guys weren't just sitting there with their heads bowed and hands folded. No, they leaped and shouted and put on quite a show. Even with all that effort being put into their prayers, however, nothing happened.

Elijah finally spoke up. I think he wanted to have a little fun at their expense as he began to taunt them. He told them to shout louder! He sarcastically suggested that perhaps their god was busy going to the bathroom or maybe he was taking a nap. When they heard that, the false prophets really stepped up their game. They shouted even louder and cut themselves with knives and swords. The crazed, bloodied idolaters continued this fruitless frenzy for the remainder of the afternoon. You can't say these guys weren't trying. They put their hearts and souls into their prayers, yet the response they got from Baal was zip, zilch, zero.

Now it was Elijah's turn. He called everyone over to watch him. He repaired the altar (as it had been torn down) and did something that I'm sure no one expected. He built a trench around the altar and commanded that four waterpots be filled with water and poured over the wood and the sacrifice on the altar. How could a wet sacrifice catch on fire? But wait—there's more! Elijah told them to do this two more times.

Just for reference, if these waterpots were the same size as the ones filled at the wedding at Cana (where Jesus turned the water into wine), each held between twenty to thirty gallons of water.[38] That means Elijah ordered somewhere between 240 and 360 gallons of

---

[38] John 2:6.

water to be poured on the sacrifice. That's about as much water as it would take to fill a four-person hot tub.

It was drenched, and the water flowed off the altar onto the ground, filling the trench. Israel had just come out of a three-year drought, so I'm sure this was no easy feat and may have aroused everyone's attention. "Hey, Uri. So Elijah is going to burn water now? Any more water and he'll need to ask God for another ark!"

Now we get to Elijah's prayer in 1 Kings 18:36b–37. "Lord God of Abraham, Isaac, and Israel, let it be known this day that You are God in Israel and I am Your servant, and that I have done all these things at Your word. Hear me, O Lord, hear me, that this people may know that You are the Lord God, and that You have turned their hearts back to You again."

That's it. No dancing, no bleeding, no shouting for hours. Just one man with a soaking-wet offering, asking God to show Himself to His people. What happened next must have made the pagan priests want to use the toilet Baal was on! As soon as Elijah was done praying, fire came down from heaven and burned up the bull, the wood it was sitting on, the stones, *and* the dust. Even the gallons of water in the trench dried up! That's some serious fire!

Both Elijah and the pagan priests had prayed. If prayer alone was powerful, the false prophets would have won, hands down. However, they were praying to a powerless, nonexistent deity. It might have made them feel better to go through all those gyrations, but what was the end result? Nothing. So it is nice when people say they are praying—I think they are being thoughtful—but in my book, it's vitally important to *whom* they are praying if you want results. When I look death in the eye, I want the assurance that I'm praying to the One in charge and that He hears me. I want to be confident that my prayers are going farther than the ceiling and are not just some psychological exercise in meditation, geared toward getting in touch with my feelings. I knew I couldn't face this alone.

So, as a believer, what *is* prayer? I was always taught, as a child, that prayer is talking to God. I also know that I don't know how to pray. There are times when I'm sick, and I can't get out much more than, "Please help me, God!" Sometimes, I have a list of people I'm asking God to protect, help, and bless. There have been prayers when I'm crying, telling Him about something hard I'm going through and pleading for direction, or when I'm asking Him to forgive me for being hurtful to another. Then there are the prayers that just praise Him for who He is. My assurance in prayer comes from this: "Likewise the Spirit also helps in our weaknesses. For we do not know what we should pray for as we ought, but the Spirit Himself makes intercession for us with groanings which cannot be uttered" (Romans 8:26–27). I imagine moments when I was in such grief that there were no words. It was then that God's Holy Spirit interceded for me. There were situations when I was uncertain *what* to pray for, and Holy Spirit interceded.

There doesn't need to be showmanship or bloodletting. I don't have to use eloquence or repetition to get His attention. Psalm 51:17 explains what God wants: "The sacrifices of God are a broken spirit, A broken and a contrite heart—These, O God, You will not despise." So it isn't always the words we say when we pray. He understands us. I believe a big part of prayer is *how* we approach Him and how our hearts respond to Him.

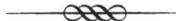

The surgery was done, and I was healing, but for some weird reason, I was itchy all over, not just where my incisions were. In addition, I felt like the area where the drain on my right side was inserted didn't want to heal. My arms still had some sores on them. I was uncomfortable. I didn't want to be touched, and I was short-tempered. Just putting on clothes activated my itching sensor.

I was feeling a bit blue, but that usually happened in autumn. So many people I know just adore "sweater weather," as they call it. People picture trees with orange, yellow, and red leaves that waft slowly down to earth, perfectly choreographed to orchestrated music.

In reality, the trees are barren, and the leaves are crunchy and brown and have slipped from the branches, unceremoniously, onto the cold, hard ground. The air is biting, and the days get shorter and shorter.

OK, does that tell you a little something about my mood? Not good. I felt like summer had passed me by and so had life. This wasn't how I was supposed to live out the last part of my youth. Well, not really youth, but soon I would hit the big six-oh, and I would be officially *old*. I had plans, and cancer wasn't one of them. I guess this was my road to Damascus. Jesus was stopping me in my tracks to put me on another course. Proverbs 3:5 tells us to let go of what we think is best and trust in God's decision and timing: "Trust in the LORD with all your heart, And lean not on your own understanding." It honors God when we yield our wills to Him, even when it's difficult, because that is what Jesus did.

It was the end of October, and although I had an invite from Rosa to go out to dinner, there was no way I was up to it. Besides, I had an appointment to see Dr. Nòvel to have my drains removed. I was anticipating a lot of pain. Just the thought of it gave me the creeps.

The doctor had offices in five locations, and up until this point, we managed to visit him at the closest locale. No such luck this time; we had to travel to what I call his froufrou office, which was over an hour away (*without* traffic, which, in New Jersey, is a rarity). This office was in a trendy SoHo-esque town. The waiting room had exposed brick on one side and nonstop windows on the other. Even the wall that encased the double entry doors was made of embossed glass. When we walked into the office, our olfactory sense was welcomed by the harmonized fragrances of freshly cut flowers and a therapeutic diffuser dispensing essential oils into the atmosphere. The bright-white atypical reception desk, with its smooth, organic shape, was a study in contrast to the distressed industrial brick walls on either side. A black-iron spiral staircase behind the desk extended up to a loft area that housed a glass-enclosed office. The cathedral ceiling, which was punctuated with oversized Edison lights, rose beyond this office on the third floor. The crowning touch was the soft, instrumental New Age music that wafted through the environment. If that doesn't say froufrou, I don't know what does.

When we were invited into the large exam room, I immediately saw the sterile stainless-steel stand with all the doctor's instruments needed to excise my drains. I quickly averted my gaze, but the only other things to see were displays that held samples of the various types of implants available. Many were quite *substantial*, and I wondered where one would find clothes to fit after having those inserted.

A tap on the door, and Dr. Nòvel entered with a nurse and a huge smile. First, Tim got a handshake, and then I received a comforting hug. He looked at me with his warm brown eyes and asked me how I was doing. I was nervous and told him so. Even though he reassured me it wouldn't hurt, I didn't believe him. Doctors *have* to say that. (But it really didn't hurt. Yay, me!)

Chapter 13

BUT WAIT! THERE'S MORE!

Remember I said oncologists don't tell you everything all at once? Well, Dr. Dawn informed me that I would be taking medicine in pill form—for five years! Ugh! On top of that, she explained that I would receive hormone treatments intravenously, so I couldn't have my port removed just yet. Before I started all this, she recommended I have a bone density test. I wish I would have had this test done *before* the chemo so I could have known with a bit of certainty what the health of my bones was to begin with.

So let's talk about this pill. The drug I was prescribed is called anastrozole, which is its generic name. It is prescribed to patients who have already gone through menopause, had early-stage cancer, and who are hormone receptor-positive. Hormone *what*? I know this is hard to grasp so I'll give you the CliffsNotes explanation.[39]

Breast cancer cells *may* have certain proteins that are receptors for

---

[39] American Cancer Society medical and editorial content team, "Breast Cancer Hormone Receptor Status," Cancer.org, last revised September 20, 2019, https://www.cancer.org/cancer/breast-cancer/understanding-a-breast-cancer-diagnosis/breast-cancer-hormone-receptor-status.html.

the hormones estrogen and/or progesterone. A receptor is a protein that can attach to substances in the blood. When the hormones estrogen and progesterone attach to these receptors, they stimulate growth, including cancer growth. If a cancer has these receptors, they are called hormone receptor-positive, or HER2-positive. In contrast, if they do not, they are referred to as hormone receptor-negative, or HER2-negative.

This medicine is an estrogen receptor modulator, which is a fancy way of saying medicine that will block estrogen. Why block estrogen? The reasoning, for many years, by the medical profession has been that if you prevent estrogen from appearing in the breast, you will also prevent cancer from reappearing, as estrogen sends out signals to grow and multiply. On the flip side, estrogen has a protective effect on bone, so precautions must be taken to safeguard yourself from osteoporosis. That's why I needed the bone scan.

I had heard about osteoporosis for many years, but I wasn't exactly sure what it was. The name *osteoporosis* literally means "porous bone." This is a disease in which the density and quality of bones diminish, and as bones become even more porous, they become fragile. With this disease, your chances of a bone fracture increase. (Well, there was one more item to put on the I-don't-want-to-think-about-it list.)

Next, I asked Dr. Dawn what she was going to put through my port this time. I just started to feel better and didn't want any more meds pumped into me. I know I drove that poor woman to tears with all my questions, but this is the only body I'll get in *this* lifetime, and I wanted to know what was going on—I think!

She told me the drugs were Herceptin[40] and Perjeta.[41] Both drugs fight cancer cells that have too many HER2 receptors[42] but each in a unique way. The possible side effects of these medications include problems with the heart. This startled me, and I asked God to protect my vital organ. I can see why people don't pester their oncologists with many questions. It's tough to ask all the questions you may have, because the answers can be so scary. It's the stuff of nightmares! I had other worries too—more surgeries, more tests, and going back to work. Would I be able to handle physical labor? I didn't know the answer to that, but I knew that once back at work, I would feel normal, and that appealed to me.

One day I read a news article about Billy Graham's daughter, Anne Graham Lotz, who had breast cancer. She was starting her chemo treatments and was losing her hair. There was a picture of her having her head shaved, and she was all smiles. This hit me. I just couldn't, for the life of me, understand why any woman would have a picture taken of this event for all the world to see. This wasn't something I wanted to share with anyone, never mind smile about it and pose for the camera. Was there something wrong with me? I hated the chemo. I hated how cancer took my breast, and the chemo took my hair. No! I couldn't smile about any of that! Just seeing that picture upset me—not because she was smiling but because I couldn't.

---

[40] Genentec USA, Inc., "Supporting You Along the Herceptin Journey," Herceptin.com, https://www.herceptin.com/?c=her-16ed7d242fa&gclid=CjwKCAjwrKr8BRB_EiwA7eFappdnXTVfORqqeLOOYGDhamGoIXsRdY3VyJkg0sbS12Ry0v9FszuGyhoCWcMQAvD_BwE&gclsrc=aw.ds.

[41] Genentec USA, Inc., "Pergeta," Pergeta, https://www.perjeta.com/patient/safety.html?c=per-16e8fec5ef8&gclid=CjwKCAjwrKr8BRB_EiwA7eFapv3G3jcK9FiYjQhhwqqOTQNdfoc6SFi5T2-Avo0D_qrjeMUXpoZU6xoCKFEQAvD_BwE&gclsrc=aw.ds.

[42] American Cancer Society medical and editorial content team, "Breast Cancer HER2 Status," Cancer.org, last revised September 20, 2019, https://www.cancer.org/cancer/breast-cancer/understanding-a-breast-cancer-diagnosis/breast-cancer-her2-status.html.

I've come to learn that we are all different. Maybe there *was* something that Anne went through that made her cry. Maybe something that didn't affect me at all had bothered her. I don't know. I am not Anne Graham Lotz; I am Adria, and God knows me and exactly what I need. That is comforting. God did that for *me*. He took me through the times where I was sad and lifted me up. He was there, protecting me and comforting me, when I was so very afraid. I sensed His peace when I had to endure pain and discomfort.

I guess what I'm trying to say is, don't compare yourself with anyone else. We all grieve differently. Our heavenly Father knows our lives are as short-lived and delicate as grass,[43] yet He loves us, cares for us deeply, and knows exactly what we need.

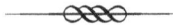

Thanksgiving came and went with all the hustle, bustle, and food prep that goes along with it. I was feeling stronger every day and was eager to start back to work and resume a more normal life. My usual custom was to put the up the Christmas tree and all the decorations on Black Friday, but I realized this would be a lot more than I could handle. Juliet and Blaise had come down for the holiday, and it was a tad too chaotic to deck the halls right then and there. One thing I have learned as the pages turn in my life is that I am mortal and can't do everything. We might not accomplish all we had planned, but that's OK. This sounds easy, but I am impatient and often must remind myself of this.

One thing I did get to do was to host a table at the annual ladies'

---

[43] As for man, his days are like grass;
As a flower of the field, so he flourishes.
For the wind passes over it, and it is gone,
And its place remembers it no more. (Psalm 103:15–16)
But the mercy of the Lord is from everlasting to everlasting
On those who fear Him,
And His righteousness to children's children. (Psalm 103:15–17)

brunch at church. The day was very festive, as we decorated tables, sang Christmas carols, and heard a message from one of us. What I mean by that is, the speaker isn't a professional; she's just ordinary folk with a message to tell. I decorated my table with a beautiful Jim Shore Holy Family sculpture that my sister had given to me. The theme was "Jesus is the Light of the World," and I accented everything with deep red and gold. I gave each woman a chocolate angel lollipop and cinnamon-scented candle, adorned with a gold bow and a scroll with Matthew 5:16 on it: "Let your light so shine before men, that they may see your good works and glorify your Father in heaven."

Everything was set and ready for the event. As I stood waiting for the ladies to arrive, I was somewhat disappointed that I didn't know any of the women sitting at my table. I was not comfortable, but I reminded myself, "Hey, I don't have cancer!" Soon, the chitchat started, and everyone was talking—but not with me. So again, I said to myself, "Hey, I'm out and about and not sick at home!"

Finally, the speaker gave us some ice-breaker activities. That's when everyone began talking, and I was able to share my experiences with them. I could see by their faces that they viewed me differently (but not with the *look*), and the walls came down. As it turned out, one of the ladies had a close relative who recently had discovered she had breast cancer. I was able to share my hope with this woman and encouraged her to be patient and keep on praying. Again, everyone handles grief differently. Her sister-in-law didn't want to be around people and wouldn't accept any help. This woman wanted to support her brother's wife, and it frustrated her greatly that she couldn't. It reminded me of a conversation I had with my mother when she got sick.

Mom had many friends who wanted to offer their aid, but she kept turning them down because she didn't want to be a bother. I explained that she needed to let people help; otherwise, she was cheating them out of a blessing. From that point on, Mom never refused people's assistance, and consequently, both parties received blessings. Sometimes it's not all about us. "Be completely humble and gentle; be patient, bearing with one another in love" (Ephesians 4:2 NIV). The day left me tired, but I was grateful. I reached out in faith, even though I was afraid, and God blessed me *and* everyone at my table.

As I began to decorate the house for Christmas, I came upon my mother's advent calendar—a small wooden representation of a plump Old Saint Nick that had twenty-five tiny pegs in his round belly. Each peg had a numbered heart that hung on it, until the twenty-fifth, which had a green holly leaf. She wasn't big on Santa Claus, but this advent calendar had been a gift, and she loved the person who gave it to her. When I opened the box to hang up the calendar, there, on the bottom of the box, was a small slip of paper with names, numbered one through twenty-five, written on it. Each time she added a heart to the jolly old elf, she would lift that person up in prayer. This touched me, and I wanted to keep up her tradition. First Thessalonians 5:17 tells us to "pray without ceasing." This little keepsake from my mother enabled me to remember people and love them in the same way that she did—by praying for them.

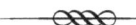

I went back to work forty-eight days after having a mastectomy. Although I was glad to be working and active, it was demanding. Each day, I would arrive home from work tired and sore. I'm sure all the walking I did helped me to grow stronger, but it was rough. When I think back, I wonder how I had the strength to do it. I wore my compression brassiere, which was hot and restricting but held everything in place and kept me from experiencing pain. I also wore my wig, and I felt beautiful!

My workdays weren't without incident, as I had some lingering effects from my treatments. One was brittle fingernails. Although at one point my nails were strong, long, and beautiful, once I stopped getting the chemo that all changed. My poor fingertips were sore because my nails were constantly breaking. Part of my job required me to replace hundreds of price labels a day. To do that I repeatedly used my fingernails. That option was no longer viable. I had bandages on my fingers and had to learn to be creative.

Another hurdle I faced was my chemo brain. Things that normally didn't bother me got my heart racing. Perhaps I'd have a conversation with someone and (in my mind) say the wrong thing. I would stew over it for days and replay the conversation in my head. I would ask myself rhetorical questions, like, "Why did I say it that way? Why didn't I shut my mouth? How come I didn't just nod my head and be done with it?" I found it helped to calm me to go back to the person and apologize. More times than not, though, the individual had to be reminded of the conversation and wasn't upset by it at all. Then, I would promptly beat myself up for being so sensitive.

My chemo brain isn't too bad now, but there are still moments when I'm having a conversation and find myself grasping for a simple word that, for the life of me, I just cannot remember. And every now and then, I still get terribly upset over a minor thing. It is on these occasions that I try to remember it's an aftereffect of my treatment and forgive myself. it sounds simple enough but takes practice.

I also found that Christmas was a good time to heal. Between the colorful decorations, joyful music, delightful seasonal scents, and planning for the big day, I couldn't help but feel happy. There was no other season like it. My hair was starting to grow in, and I was excited. Every day, I'd take off my scarf, look at my head in the mirror, and rub my hand over the soft fuzz. Because my hair was starting to grow, however, it became increasingly difficult to wear my wig. Eventually, tufts of hair stuck out from under the wig and prevented it from lying on my head correctly. I tried hard not to adjust my wig in public, as I wanted it to look natural. I've noticed that some wig-wearers tend to play with the wig, adjusting it this way and that, making it very obvious that the hair on their heads is not their own. When there's an itch that needs to be scratched, it is extremely tempting to take a pencil and stick it underneath the wig.

I seriously considered going wigless. That may sound like a no-brainer, but it was a big step for me. My new growth was only a few inches long. I felt very vulnerable, showing the world what I really looked like. I especially didn't want to expose my short, short *gray* hair! ("Woman, thy name is vanity." Despite this being a much-misquoted Shakespearean line, it is appropriate.)

That Sunday at church, I bumped into a friend I had not seen in quite a while, and we got to talking after service. She complimented my hair, not knowing it was a wig. I explained my dilemma and before you could say Jack Robinson, she said she'd color my hair for me. My eyes lit up at the prospect, and of course I agreed. So after lunch, I swallowed hard and ventured out of the house without my hair prosthesis for the very first time. I *did* wear a sweatshirt and put the hood up over my head, but after she was done, I proudly walked outside, hoodless and wigless!

As I sat facing the mirror in her home-based salon, Nurys raved about the texture, thickness, and curl of my hair. She even cut a little piece of hair off to make it even. I took the tiny curl home and placed it in my journal. I had entered her house, timid and embarrassed, but left a confident princess. If my smile were any broader, my face would have cracked.

Still, when Monday morning came, I was having second thoughts about going to work *au naturel*. Instead of giving in to my insecurities, I gathered my nerves, put on my makeup, and headed off to work, head held high. Nurys had given me a gel to hold the curls in place. I called it *snot* because that is exactly what it looked like to me, but let me tell you, that snot worked wonders!

When I walked into work, I felt exposed, but the reactions I received were positive and sincere. They weren't being complimentary just to make *the poor cancer girl* feel better. People literally stopped what they were doing to tell me I was beautiful and give me a hug. One woman I work with five days a week asked me why I kept cutting my hair. When I explained to her that I had cancer and what she had seen me with before was a wig, she was stunned. At one point, I broke down and cried. I was overcome with gratitude.

I wasn't comfortable having such a short hairdo, but evidently, I was now trendy. One of my pastors, who is African, commented, "In the black community right now, that hairstyle is very hot, and you are rockin' it!" I blushed! I also ran into Pastor Greg's wife, Lydia. She did a double-take and said, pausing between each word for effect, "You ... look ... smokin' ... hot!"

Pastor Greg didn't recognize me and told us later that he wondered who the lady was who was sitting next to Tim.

I was on cloud nine with my sassy new look but was brought back down to earth by a call from Dr. Nòvel's office. My surgery, the next phase of my reconstruction, was scheduled for March. I was afraid. I prayed and cried and confided in my three original prayer warriors. I knew I needed to *fear not* and knew, beyond a shadow of doubt, that like manna, God would provide me with everything I needed when I needed it.

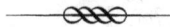

Christmas was only six days away, and there I was, back at the oncologist's office. I didn't *want* another treatment. I was just starting to feel better. I was just starting to *look* better. I didn't want to lose my hair or feel sick again.

The concern over losing my hair was unfounded because that, thankfully, was not a side effect of the medicines I was given, but feeling sick was. The following day, I had flu-like symptoms. And although my body was miserable, my heart was rejoicing. Once again, God provided comfort and shalom, shalom.

Chapter 14

OUCH TIME!

My family had busy schedules, so we decided it would be best if we all went over the river and through the woods to Pennsylvania to celebrate Christmas with Juliet and Blaise. Although I felt lousy, I was happy to be out and about. We met at a restaurant, and there were plates and food and wrapping paper all over the place. It was chaotic and a mess but absolutely wonderful. I got to hold my newest grandson and hug him till his eyes bulged out! I loved watching Blaise *ooo* and *ahhh* as he opened each of his presents. I savored every moment.

Then, a few weeks later, as was our usual custom, Christmas Eve found us at church. The sanctuary was decorated with four eight-foot trees, adorned simply but elegantly. Each was lit with hundreds of tiny white lights. Every window in the sanctuary had a navy-blue banner with a hand-painted white-and-gold dove emblazoned on it. The stage was aglow with strands of lights entwined in greenery. Gaelic music filled the air as the sound of bagpipes, tin flutes, and the traditional Irish drum, the *bodhran*, were played. The musicians and vocalists were dressed in kilts, knickers, and cable-knit sweaters as they played and sang praises to God for His blessed gift to us. I don't have to tell you that this Christmas was extra special for me.

After Pastor Greg delivered the message, the lights were turned down, and we lit our candles and sang the traditional carol *Silent Night*, the last verse a cappella. The church always looked so beautiful with hundreds of candles flickering, illuminating the darkness. At least this year, I didn't have to worry about my hair getting singed by a candle flame!

The Yule season flew by, and as we rang in the new year, I knew my surgery was soon. Being a warm-weather person, I count down the days until spring. This year, spring and my operation date coincided. Between thinking about my reconstruction and being green around the gills, it was difficult to concentrate on work. The function I perform keeps me mostly to myself. During that alone time, it was easy to allow my mind to wander, and I didn't always like where it was wandering. God's Word says we shouldn't think as the world thinks, and we need to control our thoughts. Romans 12:2 says, "And do not be conformed to this world, but be transformed by the renewing of your mind, that you may prove what is that good and acceptable and perfect will of God." How do you *do* that? I was tired, I didn't feel well, and I was frustrated. How can I change my thought pattern? I must admit that sometimes I didn't even *want to* change it. So I talked to God. I told Him how I felt, getting it all out. That included letting Him know my not-so-nice thoughts and asking for forgiveness. Just the process of doing that helped to redirect my mind, and God's power enabled me to accomplish it.

Before surgery, my temporary expander had to be inflated a little to stretch the skin. I went to see Dr. Nòvel again (at his froufrou office) and, as was his custom, he hugged me and asked how I was doing. I was nervous about having a sharp instrument jabbed into my still-sore breast, and I told him so. I soon forgot about that, however, when I found out I had to have my picture taken. Not my portrait, mind you, but one where I was mostly naked. To prepare for the reconstruction, the doctor needed to have photographs of my breasts. Before-and-after shots would document where I'd been and help the doctor and me assess the changes that were achieved. (Chances are, if you see a plastic surgeon, you will want to examine pictures of your doctor's actual patients. I guess I am now part of Dr. Nòvel's portfolio.)

The nurse directed me into a small white room. There was a tripod with a very expensive-looking camera perched on top. Silver photography umbrellas were strategically placed around the room to control the lighting. The camera was aimed at the back of the room, where I was directed to stand. This was a humiliating experience. The only fabric that covered my body were my black socks and a pair of disposable underpants that barely covered my lady parts. When I looked down, I saw what appeared to be dance-instruction footprints on the floor. (You might remember from days gone by that numbered footprints were put on the floor to indicate where beginners were to place their feet to learn the correct steps for a dance.)

For each photo I had to stand with my feet on the diagrams so I'd be pointed in the correct direction—first with my arms behind me, then outstretched. It was as if I was performing some sort of strange nude ballet. What made it even worse was that Dr. Nòvel, in his fine Park Avenue suit, was the one taking the pictures. Let me tell you—if you think you can go through all this with any amount of pride left, you are sadly mistaken.

Next, it was time to expand my implant. The doctor reassured me that it wouldn't hurt and, again, I didn't believe him. But once more, it was true. I was unsettled and looked away as he carefully inserted the needle into the valve of the expander. Before I knew it, he was done.

The next several weeks were "birthday central." Blaise, Tim, Erin, and I all celebrate during the coldest time of winter, but the constant activity helps the chilly gray days seem a little brighter. One other joyous event that took place was the removal of the port. I was elated because it meant I would no longer get any chemo!

The lump under my collarbone was purplish and uncomfortable to the touch. It reminded me of a Borg implant. The Borg are a civilization of half-mechanical, half-humanoid beings in the *Star Trek* universe. Borg is short for cyborg, and their sole purpose for being is to *perfect* all life. They achieve this by assimilating life-forms. Assimilation involves forcibly transforming individual beings into drones by injecting nanoprobes (microscopic robotic devices) into their bodies and surgically enhancing them with cybernetic components (implants). This strips them of their free will and individuality and adds the knowledge and technology of these unwilling volunteers to their own.

I felt I had no choice but to get this port implanted, and I hated it. But I, like Jean-Luc Picard, was going to be freed from the Borg Collective! (Jean-Luc is the captain of the starship *Enterprise D* in *Star Trek: The Next Generation*. At the end of season three, he was kidnapped and assimilated by the Borg. In true Hollywood style, however, by the beginning of season four, he was rescued and his implants removed.) I was going to be an individual once again!

The process to remove the port was much simpler than when it was inserted. I did not have to be sedated in an OR. Instead, the procedure was done in Dr. Nett's office, using only local anesthesia. Within about six minutes, while discussing current events, the port was removed. Although the doctor didn't say it would be, it was virtually painless. The only discomfort I felt was the injection to numb the site.

Dr. Nett's assistant cleaned off the port and gave it to me. I hated that little device, but I wanted to hold it in my hand and look at it. It was useless now. It's power to deliver any chemo to my heart was stripped from it. I was liberated! No more chemo!

The procedure was quick and easy, but I guess it was a shock to my system, and there were several days when I just did not feel well. I knew my prayer partners were constantly lifting me up, and that encouraged me. It reminded me of a passage in Exodus that told the report of a battle the Israelites had.

The Israelites were being attacked by an enemy, the Amalekites, so they went into battle against them. During this fight, Moses stood on a hilltop and raised his hands, holding up the staff of God. As long as his hands remained raised, Israel prevailed. Being human, however, Moses grew tired. He couldn't be expected to keep his hands stretched out all day. To assist him, "Aaron and Hur supported his hands, one on one side, and the other on the other side; and his hands were steady until the going down of the sun."[44] Israel won the battle. I felt like my prayer partners were holding up my hands, enabling me to win the battle over cancer.

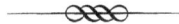

One may think that everything is in place and in order, and then *whammo*! Something happens out of the blue. I was all set to have my body put back together, and then I got a call from my insurance company that Dr. Nòvel was not covered under my plan. *I have less than two weeks to go*, I thought, *and* now *they tell me this?*

As it turned out, my company changed insurance providers, and this new insurance company didn't recognize my plastic surgeon. I didn't *want* to change doctors now. I had confidence in Dr. Nòvel. I knew I wouldn't wake up from surgery looking like the ragdoll Sally from *A Nightmare Before Christmas*. No! I didn't want to switch doctors.

During this journey, there were many detours, interruptions, and surprises when things didn't go as planned. When you are in the thick of it, it can seem like it's the end of the world. In this case, there was a lot of back-and-forth between the insurance provider, doctor's office, and me. In the end, I got to keep Dr. Nòvel.

For my mastectomy, Dr. Nòvel prescribed compression bras. For this surgery, I would need what I dubbed a *suit of armor*. It was a compression undergarment that went from below my breasts to just

---

[44] Exodus 17:12b.

above my knees. It had shoulder straps that held it up and zippers and hook-and-eye closures on both sides, from the thighs up to the underarms, to keep it in place. When I say it was tight, I mean like a second-skin tight. Also, for convenience, it had an opening in the nether region, so I didn't have to take the whole thing off every time I had to run to the little girls' room.

Suits of armor are not cheap. It wasn't a cute little pink-lace number from Victoria's Secret. This baby was tough and would hold me together! I ordered mine online, and it cost nearly two hundred dollars—you would think I *could* get it in pink for that price.

The day before surgery, I once again asked for the elders of the church to anoint me with oil and pray for me. It was peaceful. Just what I needed. My buddy Foster, who's a real tough cookie, cried for me this time.

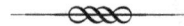

It was D-Day! I was getting my breast back. Dr. Nòvel was going to remove the extender and replace it with blood vessels, fat, and muscle from my midsection. The specific procedure I was having was called a DIEP (deep inferior epigastric perforators) flap. I tried to explain to people that it was a complicated surgery, not just filling the vacant space in my breast with fluff. It wasn't like blown insulation. I was going to be cut from hip to hip, just below the bikini line. After the skin, tissues, and blood vessels (collectively known as the *flap*) were dissected, they would be transplanted and connected to my chest using microsurgery. I found out there were to be six doctors and a doctors' assistant working on me.

In addition, I asked Dr. Nòvel to tighten up my belly while he was in there. After giving birth to three children, my midriff was a tad droopy. I didn't realize that he had intended to do that anyway. I'd read that some doctors didn't tighten up the stomach area or even perform liposuction above the belly button when performing a DIEP flap. Dr. Nòvel, however, was a perfectionist and paid as much attention to aesthetics as he did to the "meat and potatoes" of it all. His team gave me stunning results.

Dr. Nett jokingly told me that I would never have six-pack abs, as Dr. Nòvel would be using two of those muscles, and the best I could hope for were four-pack abs. I quipped that it was better than having the gallon jug that was there.

I discovered that with the DIEP flap reconstruction, no muscle was removed. I guess that Dr. Nett thought I'd be having a TRAM flap procedure, which does remove muscle.

Along with a breast, I was getting a new belly button because that part of my stomach would be removed. This didn't bother me, as my navel was crooked anyway. Earlier in my life, I'd had several laparoscopic surgeries. These types of operations are minimally invasive and involve very small incisions, one of which is in the navel. After one too many of those surgeries, my poor belly button was off center.

Dr. Nòvel thoroughly explained that after surgery, I would be monitored closely to make sure the vessels in my breast were connected and delivering blood properly. To detect this, a nurse would use Doppler ultrasound every thirty to sixty minutes. If there was inadequate blood flow, it might result in fat necrosis, which would mean the tissue had died. This then would require another surgery to remove the dead tissue. As Benjamin Franklin wrote, "An ounce of prevention is worth a pound of cure."

I was warned that the temperature of the room would be turned up to about eighty-five degrees, and I'd be enveloped in a heated blanket. However, when I woke up and saw the blanket it reminded me more of the hair dryers we had back in the sixties and seventies that had hot air blowing into a cap. Except this blower sat on the floor and I was covered in something that looked more like giant Bubble Wrap. Dr. Nòvel clarified that the heat helped the blood vessels to survive and "take" to their new environment. This didn't sound too bad to me, as I don't mind the heat, but I had no idea just how warm I would be. Also, when I was trying to fight off nausea, heat didn't help.

My surgery was scheduled for first thing in the morning, and we arrived at the hospital before sunrise. I was all clean from my dual showers with the antiseptic/antimicrobial cleanser. While I was waiting to be registered, I received a text message from one of my prayer partners. She wanted me to know she was praying for me. This dear, sweet woman set her alarm to get up before my surgery (probably around 4:00 a.m.) so she could pray for me. I was deeply touched.

Everyone at the hospital was friendly and helpful. Although it is a large facility, I wasn't just another face. Once I got signed in and received my wristband, I was brought into a small room and given instructions on how to clean myself—again. I had to repeat the cleansing routine that I'd done before my last surgery—brush my teeth with mouthwash, swab my nose, and wash down with the wipes. I can't say I wasn't nervous, but I was much calmer and happier than I was when I had faced my last surgery. I suspect it was because this time I was being put back together.

One by one, different medical professionals popped in to introduce themselves, ask questions, and jot down my answers on their clipboards. The one with whom I was most anxious to speak was the anesthesiologist. I had my little scopolamine patch stuck on behind my ear, but I wanted to make sure she knew just how susceptible I was to getting sick.

The last one to see me in the medical parade was Dr. Nòvel. Then it became more real. I was going to have this uncomfortable, misshapen, hard implant removed, and I would have *my* skin, *my* fat, *my* blood vessels in there to create *my* brand-new breast. It would be *me*!

As usual, Dr. Nòvel's face showed nothing but compassion, kindness, and understanding, all rolled up in assurance. After his customary hug for me and handshake for Tim, he sat down by my bed and pulled out a Sharpie. This sweet man was a doctor who had seen me bare more times than I could shake a stick at, but it still was embarrassing to stand there butt naked—in front of my husband, no less—and have a man draw on me with a marking pen.

It didn't take long for the nurses and orderlies to wheel me into the operating suite. I don't remember much after that until they woke me up, about six and a half hours later. My eyes were still closed, and other than being very warm, I felt rather good. Yay! There was no pain, but I felt as if I had an angry anaconda that was on fire, tightly coiled around my belly. The first thing I saw when I was brought into the recovery room, albeit very blurry, was Tim. His face was beaming.

"I feel like I've just been to church," I said, wearing my own broad smile. I did. If my hospital gown had miraculously turned into a choir robe, and I held a tambourine, I wouldn't have been surprised. I was so peaceful and happy.

I wasn't nauseated or in pain, but that soon changed. With the next shift coming on board, someone forgot to get me antinausea meds, and I started to feel sick—*really* sick. The last thing you want when you've had tummy surgery is to vomit. The head nurse was so upset when she found out. First, she chewed out the pharmacy, and then that wonderful woman stayed three hours past the end of her shift to make sure I got my meds and was all right. When the nausea subsided, I was brought into my room. The air was still, and it was hot! I love the heat, but this was ridiculous. I told the nurse I had to use the little girls' room. I didn't know I had a catheter in and was much relieved that I didn't have to get up out of bed. Sitting up was about as strenuous an exercise as I could handle.

I wanted to see what my new body looked like, so when Tim and I were alone, I pulled up my gown to inspect what Dr. Nòvel and his team had accomplished. I was afraid it would look like I had a Frankenbreast, but since Dr. Nòvel used tissue adhesive (a highfalutin medical term for glue) instead of sutures, that was not the case. My breast was nipple-less, as I knew it would be, and a flap of skin was grafted onto where my new areola and nipple would one day sit. Some women opt to have what is called a 3-D nipple tattooed onto their breasts, but I desired an honest-to-goodness, you-wouldn't-know-it-wasn't-OEM[45]-unless-you-were-my-doctor nipple.

There was a cut from hip to hip, and my new belly button was smack dab in the middle of my tummy. Even though I saw a magnificent masterpiece, I could tell by Tim's face that it was hard for him to look at me.

"He's an artiste!" I exclaimed. Which made Tim laugh and relax his grimace.

Then I noticed it. My navel wasn't round. "My bellybutton looks like a Delta shield!" I declared. For those of you unfamiliar with this, it's the Starfleet insignia that Captain Kirk has on his uniform. The geek in me was thrilled! Tim didn't believe it and got out of his chair for a closer inspection of my umbilicus. The room erupted in laughter.

Rosa stopped by to see how I had fared but had to cut her visit short. Hot flashes in an airless, overheated room is not a pretty picture. It was like putting a Klingon and a tribble in the same space. (There's a "*What?!*" Fact you'll have to look up if you don't know the reference.)

Speaking of ugly sights, the time came for me to get out of bed. Two nurses came into the room to help me move three feet from the bed to a large chair. How hard could that be? I couldn't straighten up, and I felt like my midsection had burning coals in it. The nurses locked elbows with me, got me to stand (sort of, as I was bent over like a reed in a hurricane), and lowered me into the chair. Even with pain medication, *it hurt*! I was thinking of the Wong–Baker pain scale. I would have needed one that was much larger because I think my pain level was about ninety-nine.

I wanted to be an example of a godly woman. After all, God had done so much for me throughout this journey. I wanted to show His light, even though things were not ideal. I tried to always have a

---

[45] Original equipment manufacturer.

smile on my face, say thank you, and be pleasant. But as they moved me, I was in excruciating pain. I tried not to say any expletives. Well, not only did I cuss, but I did it in two different languages. I know this might sound trivial, but I was ashamed. God had been faithful to me, and there I was, swearing. My Bible was sitting right there on the shelf for everyone to see, and I felt like a hypocrite. How could I reflect Christ? I prayed and asked God to forgive me. I cried and said, "I am so broken." I felt guilty, not so much for cursing, but I believed I had let God down. Then I heard God answer me—not verbally, but I heard Him nonetheless. He said, *I know you are broken. Everyone is broken. But I choose to do mighty works through broken people.*

Wow.

Over the next few days, the nurses helped get me to the point where I was able to walk down the hall. It was only about twenty feet, but it was a genuine accomplishment.

Every day, the nurse and I had *words*. She was trying to keep me from being in too much pain, but I kept refusing the medication. I was sure I would get sick from them. The pain was much more excruciating than the mastectomy. And contrary to popular belief, I'm not that hard-headed. I knew it was imperative I take *something* to ease the pain. Finally, we agreed on something that worked for both of us. It didn't eliminate the discomfort but made it tolerable.

After four days, I was well enough to go home. There were three drains this time—one in my breast and one in each hip.

Chapter 15

CLIMBING A MOUNTAIN IS HARD WORK, BUT WHEN YOU GET TO THE TOP, THE VIEW IS SPECTACULAR

Once again, our visiting nurse, Maria, came to our home to check my drains, incisions, and pain level. She was happy to see I was doing well and was impressed with Dr. Nòvel's handiwork. This made me happy, as I reasoned she had seen her share of recovering patients and would know good results when she saw them.

Tim was also my nurse. In addition to maneuvering me from one place to another, emptying the drains, and getting me dressed and undressed, he also applied the silicone strip to my abdominal incision. This was a delicate operation because *it hurt!* This strip was simply a length of silicone that Tim placed on my foot-long tummy wound to prevent raised scarring, or keloids. Dr. Nòvel recommended a superior-quality medical-grade silicone, as opposed to the over-the-counter brands. It was more expensive, but it was reusable and, in my opinion, worth the extra cost. There were certain things we thought we could scrimp and save on, but then, there were others, like our vitamin supplements and these strips, where the value outweighed the cost.

Sleeping was a challenge for both of us. For me, because I couldn't lie down flat, and for Tim, because anytime I needed to use the powder room, he had to get me there. Remember that I was in pain and hunched over like Quasimodo, so it wasn't an easy task. To his credit, Tim never complained and was always happy to do it.

In the back of my mind, I knew I only had three months in which to recover. How would I be able to go back to work when I couldn't even stand up straight? This surgery was not for sissies. If I had known beforehand just how painful and difficult this surgery would be, I might have thought twice about doing it. Had I gotten an implant, the whole process would have been cut short, and I would have saved myself a considerable amount of grief. I wouldn't have needed any microsurgery, liposuction, or physical therapy. It would have been over. Yes, my left breast would have been without a nipple, but the 3-D tattoo would have made it appear as though I had one. There were many times when I asked myself why I hadn't done it that way.

When weighing the pros and cons of DIEP flap versus implants, a huge pro check mark on the DIEP flap side was that once reconstruction was completed, it was done, whereas implants must be replaced. The average saline or silicone implant might last from ten to twenty years, but if there were any complications or cosmetic concerns, they might have to be changed out sooner. Did I really want to have more surgery when I was in my mid-seventies? I thought not. I also took into consideration that in the winter, regardless of whether the implants were saline or silicon, they cooled down. I had enough trouble staying warm during the colder weather, so this was a check mark on the con side for implants.

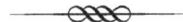

About two or three weeks after surgery, I got the bright idea to go to church. My black sweatpants and hoodie were my go-to outfit during this period. The top was loose and concealed the lumps and bumps of the drains. I was doubled over and had to walk (more like shuffle) slowly. As Tim held my arm and escorted me to my seat, someone queried if I was his mother! I was mortified, and Tim got so angry that he nearly decked the fellow. That would *not* have been a good thing to do, especially at church.

It was obvious I needed professional help to transform my backbone from a question mark to an exclamation point. Dr. Nòvel prescribed physical therapy (PT), and I was so grateful he did. In my humble opinion, everyone over the age of sixty, even if they've not had an injury, should consider having PT, just to improve their aging bodies' posture. There's a lot more to a correct stance than pulling back your shoulders and puffing out your chest. The proper carriage cuts down on the wear and tear of your joints and allows your muscles to be used more efficiently. This ultimately means less strain on your ligaments, which equals less pain. The spine is the body's structural support center. If it's not aligned properly, you *will* have problems somewhere down the line.

I began physical therapy about one month after reconstruction, and at first, it was hard and it hurt. Just walking up the six stairs to get to Dr. Pain's office was a major chore. I affectionately called her that, but Courtney was a godsend. The saying, "No pain, no gain," is spot-on. However, once I got to the other side of the discomfort and saw results, I was elated! I hope I don't sound like an egotist whose only desire was to attain the perfect body. On the contrary, my vision was to reclaim my body from cancer. For me, breast reconstruction was an important part of recovering and returning to a normal life. The blessing was that the body I got back looked and felt worlds better than the one with which I began this journey. It reminded me of Joel 22:25a—"So I will restore to you the years that the swarming locust has eaten."

Let me elaborate. Israel's crops had been destroyed by a locust invasion. When locusts destroyed crops, there were upwards of 120 million locusts covering thousands of square miles. Locusts are ravenous and destructive. Imagine the sky darkening as a swarm the size of Manhattan descends. The damage was immediate, but the impact of this devastation would be felt for years. Not only were the current season's crops destroyed, but the seeds that would generate the following year's harvest were wiped out. Grapevines and fruit trees take years to redevelop. Livestock would have nothing to eat. The entire nation's food supply could be gone, resulting in disease and economic upheaval. These people had labored in vain. All the work they had put into reaping a bountiful crop had been for naught. Loss is painful. However, God restored the years that the locusts had eaten by giving bumper harvests. "The threshing floors shall be full of grain; the vats shall overflow with wine and oil" (Joel 2:24). I felt like I had lost two years of my life. I didn't realize that God was already in the process of restoring the years that were taken from me—and then some.

My first visit to see Courtney was an evaluation. First, she asked me a series of questions that went something like this:

Q: "What are your goals?"
A: "Oh, that one is easy—to stand up straight!"
Q: "How high can you lift your leg when lying down?"
A: "Define lift."
Q: "Are you able to raise your arms up over your head?"
A: "Not even if my hair was on fire!"
Q: "Does it hurt to sit up?
A: "Is the sky blue?"

She jotted down my answers and then proceeded to work with me to see how limber I was, what my limitations were, and just which therapy would be best to get me back in shape.

Courtney was not a run-of-the-mill pretty face. If you passed her on the street, you would think she was a sweet and petite innocent young lady. Ha! That girl was as strong as an ox and tough as nails, all wrapped up in a smile and a perky little ponytail. She used that charming, soft exterior to get me up onto her torture devices, like the rack, under the guise that it was going to be fun. She didn't kid around! The next eighteen visits were filled with sweat and tears to get me to meet or exceed my goals. I hated going to PT, but I also loved it.

These ninety days of recovery were much different from my previous convalescence. I had to *work* at getting better. No lounging around this time. In between the two days a week with Courtney, I had a regimen of exercises. Some involved reaching, others utilized an oversized rubber band to stretch my muscles, and still more were just old-fashioned leg lifts, flexes, and bends. The sets were to be done three times a day and got progressively harder as the weeks went by.

I also had to massage my breast. This was not fun. When I think of a massage, I think of something soothing and relaxing. This was neither. It was more like a strong, hard jab into my sore breast. *Ouch!* My new breast was made up, in part, of fat harvested from my belly. Dr. Nòvel described the transplanted fat as a boulder that needed to be broken up into pebbles. Massaging helped with the blood flow, preventing fat necrosis, and broke up the hard lumps of fat, giving my breast a softer, more natural feel. I found it easier to do this while in the shower.

Eventually, the drains came out, and that was a milestone. Camouflaging them underneath my clothing was awkward, and I was happy to be able to wear something other than my sweatpants or extra-large flannel shirt.

People counseled me not to worry about money, that I should concentrate on getting better. But financial difficulties are not simple to ignore. Not only were the bills piling up around our ears, but to add insult to injury, there were no funds coming in. This was a huge concern. Breast cancer is expensive. My nugget of advice is to stay on top of those who control the purse strings, like the insurance company or state disability. Although they *say* they will take care of it, be a thorn in their side to *make sure* they do. Keep lots of notes with the dirty details, like names, dates, extension, and case numbers. It was during this go-round that Human Resources neglected to mail out my disability forms to the state. By the time they realized their error, an entire month had lapsed. This meant I most likely wouldn't see any income until I returned to work.

That said, we are digging ourselves out from under the mountain of invoices, but eventually, it will be paid off. With Tim's encouragement, I've tried to look at the big picture. No, there probably won't be a cruise in our near future, and I can forget about getting a new car, but I am whole.

Chapter 16

EVERYTHING OLD IS NEW AGAIN

There had been a lot of water under the bridge since I left work to begin reconstruction. To my coworkers, I had been gone three months. To me, it was eons. So much had changed. I felt like a new person, both inside and out. My goals and heart were different. Before I got cancer, I'd been looking to grow professionally, and I'd set my sights on managerial positions. Now, my spirit was more concerned with others. It's hard to explain, but some things that once were important to me were now secondary.

Sensing this, I contacted the director of ladies' ministries at our church and asked her if she needed a speaker for any event. I thought maybe there was a women's group of about ten people that might be interested in using me as a presenter for their monthly meeting. I explained what I had been through and that I desired to help others who were feeling the sting of a cancer diagnosis. Much to my surprise she asked if I would be comfortable with leading the women's Christmas brunch that year. At first, I was stunned—there would be about one hundred people there. I'm sure they wouldn't all be interested in anything I had to say. Then I thought that if I could help just one woman, I would do it. I agreed. Little did I know there would be 250 women in attendance—standing room only!

I was busy, busy, busy—working, going to PT, attending Bible study classes, writing for the brunch, and going to my frequent doctor visits. In between all this, I was working on a costume for Comic-Con and had Blaise for a weeklong visit.

Since I have a breast that's original, I must continue to get regularly scheduled mammograms. Dr. Nett said that I had a lymph node that he was "keeping an eye on." I guess he could tell by the look on my face that his comment concerned me, so he followed it up with, "It's probably nothing, but because of your history, we want to be extra careful."

This was another time when a woman might second-guess her decisions. "If I had my healthy breast removed as a preventive measure, there would be no mammograms." As it happened, there was no cause for alarm because everything was normal.

The summer soon turned into fall, and there were many days when I just didn't feel that great. The not-so-pleasant impacts of chemo persisted, and the anastrozole just didn't agree with me. My joints were achy, and I was moody. I felt as if I were getting *old* way before I was prepared to. What I mean by that is that, suddenly, I felt I couldn't do things—simple things. Going up ladders seemed rather like climbing a mountain, and kneeling became nearly impossible. Actually, kneeling down wasn't too bad; it was the getting-up part that was difficult. It reminded me of the old joke, where a man goes to see his physician and says, "Doctor, Doctor, you gotta help me. It hurts when I do this!" The doctor looks at him and says, "Well, don't do that!"

You might tell me something similar to what the doctor told his aching patient—"Stop climbing ladders and kneeling"—but I just wasn't ready to limit my mobility. I didn't want to stop doing things just because it hurt.

I was also worried about my next surgery. Almost a year to the day after my mastectomy, I would be getting my nipple and a breast lift. Dr. Nòvel was going to make "the girls" look like sisters (not twins, mind you). I was glad for this because if he didn't tweak my fifty-nine-year-old breast, it would appear that I had a granddaughter/grandma combo on my chest!

Regrettably, the weekend before my surgery I started to feel under the weather. It began with nausea and culminated in a headache so bad that I thought my skull was going to explode. Dr. Nòvel suggested we call our primary care physician, who, in turn, directed us to the ER.

Although the emergency room was packed, I was taken in right away. I held an ice pack on my head and rocked back and forth, as if that would ease the throbbing. The pain was almost to the point of being unbearable. Any worse and I think I would have passed out. I could have used that Wong-Baker scale.

The doctor quickly gave me an IV with something in it to alleviate the pain. When the pounding began to subside, a nurse came in and announced she was taking me to get an MRI of my head. As I looked at Tim, his eyes were open so wide that I thought they were going to pop out of their sockets. Yes, I was a little afraid, but I thought about the cocoon of peace. I remembered God's great works of the past.

"We know what God did last time. Let's see what He's got in store today!" I declared, and off we went to get the scan.

As I lay on the bed, face up this time, and it slowly drew me inside, I closed my eyes tightly. What I saw and heard next was mind-blowing. There was Jesus! He smiled and touched my forehead with the ring finger of His left hand and said, "I give you My peace."

This wasn't the Jesus I had always pictured. I see Him as Middle Eastern with olive-toned skin and dark-brown hair and eyes. No. He had yellow hair, and He was bright, as if light were emanating *from* Him. When I thought about it, that made sense because in Matthew 17, where Jesus was transfigured before three of His disciples, it says "His face shone like the sun, and His clothes became as white as the light." How could I be afraid when something like that happened?

As it turned out, I must have contracted some sort of virus.

Because my body was in a weakened state and in no condition to have surgery, it was postponed until the following month. I felt healthy enough for surgery that go-round. My operation was originally scheduled for 11:00 a.m., but I guess the fellow before me needed extra stitches because mine got moved to 1:45. But that poor guy must have been in dire straits because a nurse reluctantly came in and said it was now rescheduled for 3:00 p.m. I was *hungry*!

Between the waiting, lack of food, and the anxiety I naturally felt when in a hospital, I started crying when I was finally brought into the OR. Dr. Nòvel explained that many women get frightened at that point. The first surgery had been to get the cancer out. The second had been to give me my breast back. This one, however, was cosmetic. Yes, it was important—this surgery would give me a better quality of life and confidence—but could I have survived without it? Absolutely. He said it was normal to be upset, but I shouldn't worry, and that all would be well when I woke up and saw the new nipple.

Once again, Dr. McDreamy was right. When I woke up in recovery, I felt well and didn't need to stay overnight. It was pushing midnight when we left to go home.

The pain didn't kick in until two days after surgery. This time *both* breasts were sore. It was too much of a bother to take off the suit of armor, so I didn't inspect Dr. Nòvel's workmanship right away. But when the bandages came off, and I finally got a good look at what he'd done, I was amazed. I didn't know it was possible to *create* a new nipple.

At first, it was much larger than my real nipple. I didn't like it, but I could live with it. A nurse friend of mine said that she'd heard the manufactured body part would always be erect, but I found that was not the case. As time passed, and it healed and settled into its new location, it looked just like the other one—except it was white, not pink, because the skin used to create it came from my belly. Dr. Nòvel (with a twinkle in his eye) confidently said, "Don't worry; I got a guy who'll fix you right up." He was referring to his top-shelf medical tattoo artist. I must admit that I was picturing a large, hairy-armed, cigar-smoking dude named Rocco, who had tattoos on his bald head and neck, grunting, "Dere's da chart; pick a color!"

After I looked him up on the internet, it didn't matter what he looked like; his talent and professional ethics impressed me. His family worked as a team that specialized in medical tattoos.

Tattoos intrigue me, as long as they're on someone else. I like hearing the backstory of people's body art—what it means, what they were going through when they got it, things like that. I just never had the desire to get one myself. My kids were excited to hear that Mom was finally getting a tat!

While inspecting my renovated body, I was shocked to see large swaths of bruising from the lipo. In my opinion, this process of removing fat is brutal. If you've ever seen a doctor perform liposuction, it looks very violent, but that's what's required to get the job done. Large sections of my torso were the shade of ripe plums from all the pounding. I also had two cuts, about six inches long, that extended from the outside of my breast around to my back that I didn't even notice for three weeks. I was taken aback at their length but thrilled that they were barely visible (thanks to the superglue) and didn't hurt. Other than an internal stitch that took its sweet time to dissolve, my recovery was textbook.

Like last year, that summer was spent recuperating and healing, except now I was working through it. I had many days when just getting up out of bed was a laborious task, yet I think it was good for me. My pop always told me if I was hurt, I should get up and move. He felt that sitting around just made things worse. It's not easy, but anything worth fighting for usually isn't.

> I will lift up my eyes to the hills—From whence comes my help? My help comes from the Lord, Who made heaven and earth. (Psalm 121:1–2)

Along with the pain, other turbulence on this rough ride was that my insurance lapsed, and I contracted conjunctivitis (otherwise known as pink eye). It took about three weeks to get my eyes back to normal, and the insurance fiasco turned out to be a miscommunication. (Grrr!) There's nothing like being unable to see any doctors until it got straightened out. The largest pothole in the road was that the anastrozole that Dr. Dawn prescribed made me miserable. I thought I was going through "the change" *again* but much worse this time. I felt like I was about 104 years old. Not everyone has this problem. A friend of mine on this medication said she had none of these side effects. Well, at least I wasn't barking like a dog or growing hair on my tongue.

A bittersweet event was the death of Rosa's brother Angelo. His heart was damaged from previous heart attacks, and then it was discovered he had a brain tumor that needed to be removed. The mass had wrapped itself around his pituitary. This gland, which is only the size of a pea, influences nearly every part of the body, including blood pressure, bone growth, and thyroid. Without his pituitary, Angelo's blood pressure would periodically bottom out and his cholesterol hit the roof. Not a good combo when you already have problems with your ticker. I felt like someone punched me in the gut when I heard the news.

I was devastated when I lost my brother Brett on Christmas Day, 1980. He was only twenty-nine. To this day, I still weep at his passing. Rosa and I are as close as sisters. Her blood runs through my veins. If she hurts, so do I. We've been through everything together. As far as I was concerned, Angelo was my brother. I didn't want to lose him, and I agonized over it, in tears on my knees as I pleaded for my adopted sibling. Eventually, Uncle Areo, as he was called by his adoring nieces, passed away because his poor body just wasn't strong enough to fight anymore. Ironically, he went home on Christmas Eve, but not before he gave his heart to Jesus.

I'll never forget the day he was released from the hospital during the summer. The doctors had given him an abysmal diagnosis and expected him to die. This did not sit well with his wife or family members, and they told the physicians so. "Jesus is going to heal him, and he's going to walk out of this hospital," his sister-in-law declared loudly.

When Rosa and I showed up at the hospital to pay him a visit, we expected to see a comatose man, ready to cross over. Instead, we witnessed Angelo being discharged. He sat in his wheelchair, grinning from ear to ear, and waving the Bible that Tim had given to him over his head. He got up from that wheelchair on his own power and was able to get into the car by himself. Yay, God!

On a lighter note, I made it to the Philly Comic-Con with Rosa, had a wonderful (but tiring) week with Blaise, enjoyed an impromptu reunion of the Moore clan down the shore, and saw Erin graduate with her bachelor's degree. My being sick didn't make the world stop spinning. Good or bad, life goes on.

As the days began to get shorter, I realized I needed to finalize what I was going to say at the women's brunch in December. I met with Harper, the new head of women's ministries. The first thing I noticed about her was that her effervescent personality was as vibrant as her bright-red lipstick. She was young, beautiful and sharp as a tack. It was during this meeting that I found out I was scheduled to speak for thirty minutes. I like to talk, but that's a long time.

My concept was to incorporate humor and brutal honesty and convey hope to everyone in attendance. Since I was familiar with the presentation software the church uses, I went ahead and created it myself. I wanted it to end with my favorite Christmas song, "How Many Kings." The pièce de résistance would be the unwrapping of a giant Christmas present that would be on the stage behind me. I wanted the gift (which would have a large tag on it that read "To the World; From God") to be opened by children, revealing Jesus's manger. I asked Tim to help me create this vision. What I pictured was lovely in theory, but it needed quite a bit of tweaking to make it practical.

Chapter 17

WHEN THINGS GO WRONG, DON'T GO WITH THEM—ELVIS PRESLEY

There were about two weeks to go until the Christmas brunch. I was trying to remain calm and not let the little things get to me, but Tim had yet to work on the gift. We purchased what we needed to make it, but that was as far as it got. I didn't have much confidence that it would be completed on time.

Another chink in the armor was a dress I ordered. It didn't fit. Rather than get upset, I considered my options. I decided to get the dress altered and brought it to a local shop. The seamstress's first language wasn't English, so I was hoping against hope that she understood what I wanted done and that it would be ready on time. These things were out of my control, so I prayed about it and left it there. I believed the most important thing was the message. If the computer went down or the gift wasn't made or my dress didn't fit, it wouldn't matter. It was the message that would help hurting people.

It was a good thing I adopted that concept because it did not go smoothly, to say the least. My dress was finished on Friday but was still too big, so I had to use a wide belt to compensate. Then I had to scramble around on Friday afternoon to find a creche because the one I thought we could use wasn't large enough. Lastly, the gift was constructed in the wee hours before sunrise on Saturday morning—Tim had pulled an all-nighter. I could hear him in the basement, working feverishly on it when I went to bed. He was upset because he felt he'd let me down. I tried to reassure him that he had given it the old college try, and if it didn't come to fruition, it wouldn't be the end of the world. He was not convinced.

When I woke up on Saturday morning, I was excited. I put on my much-too-large dress and tried to tame my wild hair. Last year at this time, my hair was only about an inch long. Now it was thick, curly, and unruly. There wasn't much I could do but trust God for the outcome, so I headed out to church.

Tim left home before I did and had already set up the gift on stage when I arrived. In my eyes, it looked beautiful. Nancy was sitting at the controls, and she used the theatrical lighting system to illuminate the gift with red and green spotlights. The colors bounced off the silver wrapping paper, making it look like it should be sitting underneath the world's largest Christmas tree.

Unbeknownst to me, the stage was to be overflowing with teenage musicians from a local high school, who would perform Christmas carols while brunch was served. Of course, said teens decided to inspect the gift and peek under the lid to see what was inside. Some even thought it would be a good idea to lean on it, as if it were a table. They didn't realize the box was made to collapse flat to expose the real gift inside. There were a few hairy moments when I thought I was going to lose it, but in the end, I didn't kill anyone.

People were running here and there, putting the last touches on their decorated tables and greeting each other with hugs and kisses. The caterers were setting up the late morning meal, and guests were beginning to arrive. I was so excited that I couldn't wait. When the announcements, ice breakers, and games were over, it was time to eat—but I was in no condition to do so. I was wound up and anxious to get on stage. I nibbled on a few things, and then it was showtime.

A funny thing happened when I got behind the podium. As I looked out into the audience, I noticed that everything was blurry. I was concerned about using my glasses on stage because I knew I would be taking them on and off (on to read, off to look at my audience), and I thought that might be distracting. I also wanted to keep one hand on my notes (which I inadvertently put in the binder backward). I was wearing my contacts, so I should have been able to see everyone quite clearly. In contrast, without wearing what I call *cheaters* (nonprescription magnifiers), everything close to me is a blur, but when I looked at my notes, I could see them just fine. It was weird. I tried duplicating the phenomenon the next day, just to determine what had happened, but I couldn't.

I took a deep breath, put my glasses down, and held my head up. I tried to remember everything I had learned in drama class—speak clearly and loudly, look at your audience, be animated to make a point, smile, and if you have to pee, use it! (That last one is a reference to always having to run to the john at the last moment and not being able to because you'll miss your cue. So if you must *go* that badly, use that urge to give the best performance you can.)

I honestly felt like I was speaking to a room full of friends. I knew many of these ladies and the others were friends I just hadn't yet met. I had confidence that God was working, and it was exhilarating. I told them about the cancer, the MRI, and my fears. But I emphasized, with tears, that through it all, God was there. He cares and loves us so very, very much. "How much?" I asked. "This much!" And I spread my arms out as wide as I could.

Behind me on the screen was a picture of our Lord on the cross. I stepped to the side, out of sight, and the lights went dim. Two women then went on stage and took the lid off the gift so the sides fell open, revealing the manger inside. Next, the video of "How Many Kings" was played.

At least that was what was *supposed* to have happened. What actually occurred was kind of amusing in retrospect. Tim had been so worried that the gift would fall apart or open prematurely that he might have secured it a little too tightly. However, one swift kick convinced the stubborn side to open. Alas, the creche wasn't elevated high enough, so the people in the back of the room couldn't see it; the poinsettias lining the front of the stage were probably blocking it from view anyway. Then, after the gift's grand opening, we all sat in the dark for a moment (it felt more like hours). The women didn't know anything else was going to happen and began talking among themselves, and *then* the video started.

I can't lie; I was disappointed. That's not how I had envisioned it. Regardless, I know everything we did that day made a difference. A number of women came up to me afterward with heartfelt thanks. One was recently diagnosed with cancer and shared how scared she was. I was able to cry with her and offer my help and prayers. Another approached me with her mother, who had gone through breast cancer. She had been her mom's caregiver and was so thankful I was telling the story of the support person's plight as well. I was humbled and grateful that my mess was turned into a message to help those who were scared and hurting. Had I not had cancer or gone through any of this heartache I wouldn't have been able to do that.

> Blessed be the God and Father of our Lord Jesus Christ, the Father of mercies and God of all comfort, who comforts us in all our tribulation, that we may be able to comfort those who are in any trouble, with the comfort with which we ourselves are comforted by God.
>
> —2 Corinthians 1:3–4

Chapter 18

OUT OF THE BLUE

Dr. Nòvel had examined me and just wasn't happy with what he saw. He wanted to tweak my left breast just a little. He said he wasn't satisfied with the shape of my areola and explained that even a tattoo would not hide the imperfection.

I thought about having another surgery and wasn't too keen on the idea. But then I thought about how far I had already come; I didn't want to stop prematurely. The areola was larger and more oblong than it should have been. The operation shouldn't be that much of a to-do, I reasoned. It wouldn't require an overnight stay at the hospital or general anesthesia. I would be given twilight sleep. So I agreed to have the touch-up, and my surgery was scheduled for March 2020.

By now, everyone knows what was going on at that time. Just about the whole world was under quarantine because of COVID-19. So my operation was put on hold indefinitely. It seemed as if the entire human race was doomed, but I knew better. I read the Book, and I know how it ends.

Businesses were closing, and people were isolating themselves. I started to worry about what we would do if my company closed its doors. How would we survive? I knew I had to trust God for whatever came our way. I didn't realize it at the time, but my business was considered essential, so I was never out of work. While most people were suffering from severe cabin fever because they were stuck in the house, I was at the opposite end of the spectrum and would have loved to spend a day or two home in my pj's. I was one of a handful of people willing to venture out to physically go to work. The hours were longer and extremely hard. Under normal conditions, I would have been tired, but with the aftereffects of chemo, let's just say I was in a perpetual state of exhaustion.

I understood why the powers that be considered a hardware store essential. If your water heater blew up or your basement flooded, and you required supplies to remedy the situation, that would be essential. I got it. But that's not why folks were flocking to the store. The busiest departments were paint and garden. (I don't think varnish or a lawn mower are vital to one's survival, unless you're MacGyver.)

About 75 percent of my coworkers were self-quarantining. The skeleton crew that was left became experts in everything. There wasn't a job in the place that we didn't do. On top of that, we endured a fair share of abuse. Customers were lined up at the door, waiting to get in to get their *essential* mulch, paint, and patio furniture. That line sometimes extended one hundred feet away from the front door, so they weren't always in the best of moods. None of them wanted to hear that there wasn't anyone available to operate a forklift to get their firepit down from the overhead. One man I attempted to assist got furious with me that there were no kitchen designer experts on duty. Online orders were so backed up that a job that normally took two people now required a staff of fifteen to twenty. Whole aisles were closed, as they were chock-full of shopping carts containing the products people purchased from the comfort of their homes. We had nowhere else to store the items that were waiting to be picked up curbside. And, as you may surmise by that last comment, there were scant few carts for the in-person customers. In addition, each shopping cart had to be disinfected after every use. That all took time, and most of the patrons didn't like the inconvenience.

We were frontline workers, taking all the risks that the quarantined people were avoiding, but I guess they never thought about us. We were the people who stocked, packed, and rang up all the things they *needed* to prevent boredom. We were tired, dirty, and felt underappreciated. In all honesty, some folks definitely needed an essential item, but to us, they seemed few and far between.

I wasn't afraid, but there were plenty of people who were. We saw them, day in and day out, wearing all kinds of PPE (personal protective equipment). One woman (at least, I thought she was a female; I wasn't sure because she more closely resembled a space alien) wore a cleanroom suit with her gloves duct taped on, goggles, a face mask, and a shield. Our everyday jobs were twice as stressful because we were bombarded with a daily dose of doom and gloom by the news outlets. Every day they warned us that death was at our door.

Part of my daily routine was to disinfect everything my team touched—every two hours. That meant toolboxes, printers, ladders, phones, doorknobs, and hammers. Trying to keep a six-foot distance from others was nearly impossible. Customers tended to come right up to us and remove their masks to talk. They felt they couldn't be heard through the thin cloth, so rather than just speak louder, they'd take them off. We managed to do it, though, and by the time we punched out to go home, some of us were hoarse from yelling through masks and Plexiglas for the entire day.

To keep a healthy space between others, I often felt like I was playing a weird game of Mother, May I. While walking at a brisk clip, I'd suddenly stop short when coming toward others. Next, after confirming who would go first, we would zigzag around to avoid contact. When there was a group of people, it was more like the child's game Red Light, Green Light. We'd all freeze in our steps;

then, one at a time, each one would take halted steps in different directions until everyone was a safe distance away.

My heart went out to the individuals who were sincerely afraid. I could see it in their eyes. It made me sad. Then there were those who took advantage of the situation. For instance, individuals couldn't come to work because they feared for their health, but they had no qualms about showing up as a customer for obviously nonessential products.

It was an incredibly taxing time. Don't get me wrong; I was grateful I was working. So many businesses were closed that the large strip mall in which our store was located looked like a ghost town. People couldn't feed their families, as there just wasn't any money coming in. Food pantries were running out of supplies, and the fear factor was off the scale. Yes, I was grateful, but it didn't relieve the tension I felt daily. There was unlimited overtime, and when I was able, I was there six days a week. I did my best but had to realize my limitations. I, like many of my coworkers, was worn-out, irritated, and tense.

I usually wrote something for this book every day. I'd heard that's how John Grisham penned his first manuscript. He was a lawyer and family man and served in the state legislature, but he always made time to write every day, no matter how tired he was. It took him three years to complete his first book, but he did it. I tried to adopt his practice, but during this chaos, I completely stopped. I was drained and couldn't concentrate. As usual, God had different plans for me.

Although our church building was shut down, we continued business as usual with online services. We try to keep up-to-date with the latest technology and had a plethora of resources to make this happen. Before the unleashing of the coronavirus, we were already hosting live Facebook events, so we were somewhat prepared. It was exciting, as it reminded me of the early church. People of the Way were on fire for the Lord. And although they were persecuted and had to flee their homes, God turned a bad thing into something good—the gospel was spreading!

The physical church doors may have been closed, but the church (His body of believers) was very much alive and well and at work. All over the world, tech teams sprang into action to bring the good news to the airwaves and the World Wide Web like never before. I believe spiritually hungry people were ready and waiting to hear about something, some *one*, who would give them hope. I say that, in part, because our congregation had about one thousand attendees on Sundays before the virus. Now, with the online services on Facebook, our website, and YouTube, twice that amount were tuning in.

We were in the middle of a sermon series from the book of Zechariah called Unquenchable Hope. These sermons were planned out in advance, so it wasn't intentional to have this hope-filled series during a hopeless time—at least, not by the pastoral staff. However, these faithful servants seek God's providence in all they teach, so it wasn't the first time a sermon was about just the right thing at just the right time. I knew it wouldn't be the last either.

Zechariah was a prophet of God who was among the Jews who were permitted to return to Israel after their seventy-year exile in Babylon (present-day Iraq). Their first act upon coming home was to rebuild the temple that had been destroyed. Our pastor encouraged us to press on and, regardless of the chaos around us, strive to do whatever task God had us do. This struck a chord with me. I had put off writing because my mind was elsewhere, and my body was beat up. I didn't think I could compose anything worth reading. Then, I remembered Nehemiah, who was born during this exile and was a cupbearer for the king. Although he had never even been to Israel, Nehemiah had a burning desire to rebuild the wall around Jerusalem. But what could he do? He was only a servant and not even physically present in Israel. His first action (and a wise one, I might add) was to seek God's intervention by praying and fasting, and Jehovah-Jireh made a way. Not only was he granted permission to go to Israel, but the king gave him supplies and protection. The

Jews had enemies who didn't want to see the wall reconstructed, and they tried to prevent it by whatever means possible, including deception and murder.

Through the leadership of Nehemiah, work on the wall began and was done by everyone. Families, priests, artisans, men, and women all participated. They didn't let their enemies stop them from doing God's work. Swords were worn at their sides, and some did their work with one hand, while holding a weapon in the other.[46]

I thought I could write while holding a weapon. God would provide for me too.

---

[46] Nehemiah 1–4.

Chapter 19

THE DIFFERENCE BETWEEN SOMETHING GOOD AND SOMETHING GREAT IS ATTENTION TO DETAILS—CHARLES R. SWINDOLL

After the pandemonium that ensued from March through June, many believed it was now safe to emerge back into society. St. Sebastian's Hospital must have thought so too because it was now allowing elective surgery (although abortions were never banned in New Jersey during this time),[47] and I was scheduled to go under the knife again.

Once more, I had to wash with Hibiclens, swab out my nose with gook, and starve to death as I waited an additional three hours to have my chassis straightened out. And again, I kicked myself for agreeing to more surgery. I saw the big picture, but I was tiring of the procedures to get there. Everything had been drawn out way too long. In hindsight, it wasn't a rough recovery, and I was able to

---

[47] New Jersey Gov. Phil Murphy's (D) Executive Order 109, March 23, 2020, https://nj.gov/infobank/eo/056murphy/pdf/EO-109.pdf.

go back to work right away with few restrictions, but I was growing weary.

The only item left on my to-do list of getting *me* back was to inject a little color into my pasty-looking parts. Since I had never had a tattoo, I didn't know much about the procedure. I asked a few people questions, but their tattoos were on their arms, backs, or legs. Mine would be on a very delicate part of my anatomy, and although I was still numb in spots from the surgeries, I had some feeling in my breast and wasn't looking forward to a needle (even a tiny one) being repeatedly stuck into it.

My last appointment to see Dr. Nòvel put my mind at ease about getting colorized. We were just about the only ones there because the COVID-19 restrictions were still in place. And because of those constraints, I couldn't give him the biggest hug in the history of the world. I was so used to getting a warm embrace from Dr. Nòvel each time I saw him, but now, when I wanted to express my appreciation with all my heart, I couldn't. I tried telling him how grateful I was, but the KN95 face mask I was wearing fogged up my glasses and made it difficult to speak. I felt like such a dork. However, he appeared to be touched by my feeble attempts to thank him and said he was happy that everything had worked out.

I didn't realize just how excited I was. For once in my life, I didn't look back and regret my choices. Since I didn't have implants, I wouldn't need any revisions or replacements.

After the exam, I had to go into the white room and perform pirouettes before the camera one more time, as Victor Mann, the medical tattoo artist, needed up-to-date photos. As embarrassing as this process was, I would not object to showing a prospective patient the impressive results I received from Dr. Nòvel and his team. If it means giving a fellow member of Team C a glimmer of hope, I am all for it.

Victor's goal was to make medical tattooing an integral part of the reconstructive process. He wasn't an amateur who decided to do this just to make extra cash. He was an experienced tradesman in the field of tattooing and used traditional tattoo pigments and machines, which means his procedure was permanent. Doctors sometimes make use of support staff for this step. These individuals, although trained, may have little experience in actually applying tattoos. Victor was dedicated, internationally known, and in high demand. As a courtesy and to give his patients the best of the best, Dr. Nòvel had an arrangement with Victor to travel to New Jersey just about every quarter.

Leading up to the visit, I was delighted that this last step was going to be over soon. I was highly disappointed, however, when I learned that Tim couldn't come into the office with me. As it turned out, the Hoboken office was on the petite side. Since there was still a coronavirus restriction in place, I understood why they needed to limit the number of people in the office. I also remembered how hard it was to thank Dr. Nòvel while wearing a face mask. Since I would have to wear one the entire time, I decided to use it to help me show my gratitude. With a blue marker, I wrote, "Thank you, Dr. Nòvel and Victor Mann," across the front of it.

The office was on the top floor of a medical building, nestled between a bank and a traditional brick-faced apartment building, which I'm sure had been converted into condos. Although only seven stories high, it was taller than most of the other buildings on the block. When I opened the door to the office, I was taken aback by its sterility. What I mean by that is that everything was white. If it wasn't white, it was chrome. Although the eastern and southern sides of the room were floor-to-ceiling windows with an unobstructed view of the New York City skyline, it was all too plain (and trendy) for this country girl. I wanted colorful balloons and confetti to drop from the ceiling! I expected everyone there to be just as excited as I was, but the mood in the nearly silent room was as stark as its decor. I uncharacteristically took a few selfies. But before I did, I was careful to turn the sound off, as I knew it would ricochet off the walls and draw attention to my awkward attempts to capture the Freedom Tower over my left shoulder.

A few minutes later, I was directed into an even smaller white room. After disrobing and covering myself with a blue paper sheet, of sorts, Victor entered, greeted me, and began the process. I knew who he was as soon as he walked into the room because I had seen news videos that highlighted Victor and his altruistic work. I especially recognized his porkpie hat.

It was originally planned that I would get only my rebuilt breast tattooed, but since my right nipple was very pale, he colorized both to have the shades more synchronous and natural. I didn't have much feeling yet on my left side, so numbing cream wasn't needed. He applied quite a bit to my right side, however, and I certainly was glad he did. It didn't hurt as bad as I thought it might, but it wasn't something I'd go out of my way to feel either.

As he worked, we made small talk about our grandchildren and Victor's first tattoo, some thirty-five years ago. It didn't take long before we made the connection that although we lived in different states, we both lived in the *sticks*. I got the feeling that this city setting was a tad too froufrou for him as well.

The process didn't take long, and I was sent home with a pink bag that contained all I needed to care for my sore, bandaged sisters. *Very uneventful*, I thought. Despite some itchiness and tenderness for a few days, it wasn't too bad.

With all this behind me, I could look in the mirror and love the reflection. I was done. I had *me* back. Reconstruction was more difficult than I had imagined, but the results were amazing. Nurses have asked me which breast was the one removed because they can't tell. It's not like I'm going to appear in some girly magazine or even wear a bikini, for that matter, but I feel fabulous in my own skin. The best news for me, though, was that throughout this entire process, God kept His word. It was a long and winding, hilly road to travel, but I was never alone.

Now, at the end of this road, I am all right. Yes, I tire more easily, and I have a few more wrinkles than when I started, but my heart is glad.

The LORD is my strength and my shield; My heart trusted in Him, and I am helped; Therefore my heart greatly rejoices, And with my song I will praise Him.

—Psalm 28:7

Chapter 20

SOME SUPERHEROES DON'T WEAR CAPES

Superman once said, "I think a hero is an ordinary individual who finds the strength to persevere and endure in spite of overwhelming obstacles." In my opinion, this describes caregivers. They don't *have* to be in the middle of all this cancer nonsense, but they are. I saw my Tim like Superman—unassuming, selfless, tenacious, and lonely. The bullets that were shot at him bounced off his chest. You would never know that deep down inside, he hurt, and he wanted this to be over. He put on a strong face, but he was more afraid than I. When he looked in the mirror, he saw mild-mannered Clark Kent, who was weak and couldn't fight off a cold, never mind villains. But I saw the Man of Steel.

I saw someone who loved me and still called me beautiful, even when I was bald and covered in sores; someone who never complained and cheerfully did whatever he could to make my life just a little easier. If it meant massaging my aching feet, cleaning up after I vomited, or changing soiled sheets in the middle of the night, he would do it. Maybe I was the one with the x-ray vision because I saw beneath his tough exterior into his heart. He was willing to give me his last breath if it meant I didn't have to suffer anymore. Even though he didn't wear a cape, Tim was my superhero.

I decided that I wanted to delve into what caregivers go through. I knew what I had to endure, but I wanted to take an unfiltered look into caregivers' souls. I realized it might be beneficial to interview other caregivers, both male and female, to get their perspective. (Note: I did not sugar-coat their responses, and their names have been changed to protect their anonymity.) The purpose of this exercise is to give insight into what a caregiver experiences and perhaps lend a hand to one who is struggling to manage this colossal responsibility.

The superheroes I interviewed were:

Betty, who cared for her mother for four years as she suffered from liver cancer. Her mother was under treatment to eradicate three tumors before she was eligible for a transplant. Sadly, she died during treatment without ever receiving the transplant.

Fred, who was newly married when his wife was diagnosed with breast cancer. They had no children living with them. His wife has since recovered and is healthy.

Wilma, whose mother had three bouts with breast cancer—the first in her left breast in 1999 and the second in her right breast, six months after finishing her first cancer treatment. The third diagnosis was made in 2008. The first two were treated with a lumpectomy, removal of lymph nodes, and radiation. She had a double mastectomy with no reconstruction when it was determined she had breast cancer for a third time. She is currently healthy, retired, and living with Wilma.

And last, *Barney*, who cared for his wife when she was diagnosed with acute myelogenous leukemia (AML). She stayed in the hospital for nearly six months. While there, she had an accidental fall that resulted in a brain bleed and was in a coma for five days. They had two teenage children at the time. Barney's wife has since recovered, and the two enjoy doting over their grandchildren.

- Did you have a job while you were caring for your sick loved one? If so, how did you handle it?

Betty: I was working, but it was not full time, and I had flexible hours. My father worked, and he had the benefits. My dad provided everything she needed physically—insurance, a roof over her head, and food. It was never discussed who would take care of her. It just happened that I would be the one to stay home and care for my mother. My dad never verbally told me, but his eyes said, "My daughter, I'm sorry that you have to go through this."

Fred: No. I think one of the things that helped me was that I knew I could be single-focused on full-time caring, if it came to that, because I didn't have a job. This [caregiving] became the priority. Everything else could roll to the side because I didn't have to beat the reaper with a nine-to-five job. It was a blessing in terms of the timing.

Wilma: When she had her double mastectomy, I was currently off from work because I was recovering from surgery on my feet. The timing was really good. Since she didn't have chemo, she wasn't really sick. I took care of her drains. I monitored and measured them and helped her with the dressings. It wasn't much. She was limited, but she did fine. She was slowly moving her arms and raising her arms and then, I think, slowly carrying things, depending upon their weight. She was functional. The first two times she had cancer, she had a lumpectomy and radiation, no chemo. Mom drove herself to radiation and was well enough to go to work, so this wasn't an issue for me. But it was only really the third time, when she had the mastectomies, that I had to help her a bit. It wasn't a tremendous amount.

Barney: I was self-employed, doing home improvement, and the day after she was diagnosed, I quit working. I spent five and a half months in the hospital with her. I slept in a chair. Financially, we were hurting. We took out a catastrophic health insurance plan right before this so that paid for the big stuff. But the co-pays and other expenses added up, and we ended up losing our house over it. It went into foreclosure.

- What was your reaction when you found out your loved one had cancer?

Betty: We were in the doctor's office with my aunt when he told my mother she had cancer, which I call the monster. My mother looked like a zombie when she heard the news. Then she broke down and cried. My aunt was crying. But at that moment, I was trying to be positive and strong for my mother. I heard what the reality was and what the doctor said, but I thought, *There is God, and He is big and good*. I chose to take the path of believing in God to do a miracle. Sometimes in life, you will come face-to-face with news, and instead of crying, we have to find a solution or a way to do the immediate—fix it or deal with it. Reasons or consequences we can deal with later. I visualize things. I took the road of God, hope, treatments, options, doctors' opinions, and choosing to be positive and hopeful.

Fred: I didn't know enough about it [cancer] to be fearful or worried. It's like it's the first time something touches your family. I never had an experience when cancer touched my family, that I can think of. I wasn't comfortably numb, but I didn't have a panicked reaction either. I was concerned about how my wife was going to respond. I was just gutting it to get through it. I don't recall the bad stuff. My mind doesn't remember the bad stuff. Maybe I blocked it out. I don't relate on a feelings level. When I'm in rough circumstances or pressure is building, my comfort is to create order out of things—routine, mundane things. It helps me to cope with the pressures of the circumstances. It became more acute. I knew there were things that I would have to do to ease her burden. I didn't want her to have to do laundry. I didn't want her to have to worry about stuff in the house. I wanted her to be comfortable. Some spouses—well, really, the husband—can deny their feelings. They are focused on their job. Some guys shut down so much, that all of a sudden, their spouse becomes unattractive, and they leave. I would have to say that I wasn't having that sense or feeling, but I didn't want to think it could be any worse. I didn't think it was unto death. My mind didn't go there. I just knew it was going to be a bumpy ride for a while. I resigned myself to thinking long term. I remember feeling inadequate. When I helped her, I helped me.

Note: In hearing Fred's statement, I looked up some statistics on this and found out that Fred's reaction is similar to many husbands who find themselves in this position. According to a study by Mijung Park, PhD, MPH, RN, published in the *American Journal of Geriatric Psychiatry*, there is a difference in how men and women approach caregiving. It seems that men more frequently focus on tasks and to-do lists. They also will not hesitate to hire someone to assist them. Whereas women in the caregiver role may need more support emotionally.[48]

In addition, and most unfortunately, Fred was not wrong in his statement about husbands leaving their wives. Another study, which can be found in the National Library of Medicine, National Center for Biotechnology Information, indicates that when a wife gets a serious illness, such as brain cancer or multiple sclerosis, she is six times more likely to be abandoned by her husband after a diagnosis.[49]

Wilma: My mother told me. I'll never forget the first time she had cancer. It was 1999. I was out of college and working. I was away in Upstate New York for a winter weekend at Camp of the Woods. I

---

[48] M. Park, "In Sickness and in Health: Spousal Caregivers and The Correlates of Caregiver Outcomes," *American Journal of Geriatric Psychiatry* 25, no. 19 (2017):1094–1096, doi:10.1016/j.jagp.2017.07.004,
https://www.ncbi.nlm.nih.gov/pmc/articles/PMC5785240.

[49] MJ Glantz, MC Chamberlain, Q. Liu, CC Hsieh, KR Edwards, A. Van Horn, L. Recht, "Gender Disparity in the Rate of Partner Abandonment in Patients with Serious Medical Illness, Cancer," 115, no. 22 (Nov 15, 2009):5237–42, doi: 10.1002/cncr.24577. PMID: 19645027, https://pubmed.ncbi.nlm.nih.gov/19645027.

was talking to her on a pay phone when she told me. I started crying, and I felt bad because I was so far away from home. I cried a lot and told my friends who were there, and they prayed with me.

Barney: She went to the general practitioner for blood work because she was tired all the time. He told us she had something called leukemia. But when we saw the oncologist, he said the type of leukemia she had was fast-moving but the most curable. I was devastated. No one I knew who had this survived. I thought I was losing my wife. I couldn't handle it.

When she went into the hospital, I told the kids we would be there overnight, but she didn't come home for five and a half months. The hospital did allow her to come home for three days at Christmas, but then she had to go right back in. I was with her for five and a half months. I only ran home to change clothes. The kids took care of themselves, but eventually my in-laws moved in and took care of the kids.

- How did you handle telling other family members the bad news (repeating the information and answering the same questions over and over)?

Betty: My family lives in another country. My mother called and told her family. She broke the news; they cried, and then I would talk to them. Even though they are far away, speaking with our family made us feel like my dad and I were not alone. This was before cell phones and Facebook, so we bought my mother a lot of calling cards so she could speak to her family, and they cried, mostly, but I think it helped to communicate with each other.

I had to tell my younger brother. He got really worried and asked a lot of questions. I let him know everything I knew. I think, in the beginning, he was in shock. He couldn't believe it. It wasn't until right before she died that he finally realized this was real.

Fred: I didn't tell her family; she did. I didn't know enough about it to talk about it. When I did speak to them to keep them updated, I was being pumped with questions, and I didn't know how to answer them.

Wilma: My mother told everyone. So I don't know how it went down.

Barney: I only told my brother because that's the only other family I had. She told the kids, and I went into the woods and cried.

- Did any family members handle the news badly? If so, what happened?

Betty: My one aunt, who was older than my mother, took it bad. When my mother was little, my aunt used to protect her like a mother. After she heard the news, she cried a lot and was not eating well.

Fred: No. There was concern. No emotional outbursts. My sister showed the most concern.

Wilma: I don't remember how it went down with my grandmother the first two times. She was always a big worrier, a big worry wart. She would be consumed with worry. I do remember the third time, though; when Mom was getting the double mastectomy, she didn't tell my grandmother. She decided to tell her after it was all done because she knew my grandmother would be an emotional wreck.

Barney: My seventeen-year-old daughter did, but she covered it up. She put on a good face for me, but she was struggling a lot. She couldn't handle seeing her mom bald. It upset her greatly, and my wife had to get a wig. My fourteen-year-old son didn't realize how serious it was until he got older. My wife's two brothers were very understanding. They even knew a specialist who looked over all her results and gave us his opinion. That was very encouraging. Everyone thought we should be in Sloan Kettering and gave us a hard time about that, but it happened fast, and we wound up somewhere else. That was good because that doctor saved her life. I'm convinced of that.

- Did you find yourself having the same symptoms as the person who was ill (sympathy pains)?

Betty: No. It killed me to see what my mother was going through. I wished I could change places with her. If I could have, I would have given her my arm so she wouldn't feel anything.

Fred: As it got deeper into the treatment, I did. There was dizziness—vertigo. There were a couple of things, but I don't remember. I was picking up on my wife's discomfort. I was picking up on what she was going through.

Wilma: No, but I remember sitting in the recovery room with her after she had the mastectomies. Her chest was bound, and she had drains. When I sat there, I felt a sadness that she lost her womanhood; she was disfigured and not physically the same anymore. For a while, when I first started seeing her without her dressing, and she had her staple line across her chest, it was sad. She was disfigured and wasn't the same. Talking about it now makes me well up, thinking about it. Even after the scar healed and I saw her chest—you can see the sternum and ribs underneath. It cut my heart a little bit, realizing how she had been affected like this. Her body wasn't the same. I don't think I ever admitted that to her. It took a while to get used to how her body looked. I would feel sad. Today, I'm fine with it, but every once in a while, I'll feel a little stab to my heart. I have to remind myself that even though she may not have her breasts, at least I have my mom.

Barney: No. I've heard that sometimes happens, but I didn't experience that. Her biggest symptom was she was exhausted.

- If you could travel back in time and come face-to-face with yourself, what is one piece of advice the you of today would tell the you of yesterday?

Betty: You are strong, even though you don't know it yet. In the end, you'll be OK, even though you don't feel like it.

Fred: Just to mentally be prepared for the long haul. We think when someone's ill, they'll be sick for a few weeks, and it will be done. But this wasn't the case. There were months with doctors' appointments and adjustments to medication and adjustments to surgeries, witnessing the pain and discomfort. You need to have an attitude of just doing the next thing or handling the next circumstance with patience and perseverance. And as often as you think about it, give it up to the Lord.

Wilma: I don't remember how I felt while my mom was being treated. It was just kind of mundane. It didn't seem like a big deal because she wasn't incapacitated. She wasn't really physically affected. If it had been more dramatic, if things were worse for her, or if she was in a worse condition that required more of me, I might have a different answer.

Barney: It would be to say, "Be more sensitive to your children and their feelings." I don't think I would change anything else. I would still stay in the hospital with her.

- What did you do to motivate yourself during dry times?

Betty: I didn't have time to think about me. My aunts say that I devoted myself 100 percent to Mommy and that there was nothing else in my mind. I didn't think so at the time, but now I do.

Fred: I think I read the book *Unbroken* in the beginning. It's an amazing story of a very self-determined man and athlete who breaks a world record in track and volunteers as an airman at the beginning of WWII. It's his story of fierce determination to survive a crash landing in the sea, record [number] of days adrift [at sea] with two other men, being captured by Japanese navy, and imprisoned for the remainder of the war in multiple horrid prisoner-of-war camps. He became motivated by hatred. But God in His grace reached him when the war was over. He was a broken man, consumed with alcohol dependency, hatred, and revenge. He responded to a Billy Graham call to repentance, and his life radically changed, with God replacing the hatred and the nightmares with perfect peace and a determination to go on to the ripe age of ninety-four. He served the Lord by serving others, particularly young, troubled boys and girls from the inner cities. It helped to encourage me about endurance. I was impressed with how much these guys had to endure, which made my situation pale.

Wilma: I don't know. As a critical care nurse, the staff might look at a patient, and we just know he/she is going to die. It's hard for us to see patients suffering so much, and then the things we do to them and for them [to help them get better] only causes more discomfort and pain. For health care workers, that's called moral distress. We see them suffering, and we feel we are adding to it, as well as prolonging it. To be honest, we'll think that the family should let him go and end his suffering, but of course, we don't tell them that. I have to check myself and my thoughts and remember to be more understanding that the family doesn't want to give up on their loved one. I try to put myself in their position, especially when the family is making the decision to let their loved one go. Unfortunately, I've been a part of those moments many times, and it grieves me to see what those families are going through. I am very cognizant of the fact that this family is going to remember their loved one's death for the rest of their lives. And part of that memory will include the nurse that cared for him/her. With that in mind, I've got to be on my toes. I am caring for the patient but caring for the family as well. I thank God that I have never had to make the decision that they are making, and I pray I never will. But I imagine myself in their shoes, and then I cry with them.

Barney: I'm not sure. I thought about how God had brought us through with miracles, and I prayed. I told myself I didn't have a choice; I had to keep going.

- Did you ever get angry at your loved one, simply because they were sick?

Betty: No. A few times I got mad but not at her. I would get mad at others at how they treated her. I wouldn't say anything, but I would react. I had body language that showed I was angry; I'd make faces or huff and puff or slam doors. My mother would apologize to me because she felt bad that I was being her witness [her caregiver] and that it was her fault she got sick. But I would tell her she didn't have to apologize, and it wasn't her fault. I would tell her, "You didn't ask for it." Mommy said I was missing my life. But I would not be anywhere else. She was my mom. Where else would I be?

Also, a doctor explained to me that my mother had a very low tolerance for pain. Just getting a needle would cause her to scream. I didn't understand this until the doctor explained it to me. She was afraid of needles and hospitals. She worried more about what was going to happen to her [CT scans, needles, etc.] than the cancer. Someone asked me if I would be my mother's witness again. Yes. I would be her arms and legs and do it all over again.

Fred: Yes. Sometimes things were inconvenient. I wanted it my way, and I couldn't do it. I had frustration over not being able to fix it, make it go away. I also missed intimacy. That created stress.

Wilma: No because we assumed it was because of the hormone replacement. She had been smoking cigarettes all throughout this time, from the first diagnosis to the third, and the doctor said he didn't think it was a contributor to her breast cancer. We thought she got cancer from hormone replacement during menopause. She was sold on the idea of hormone replacement. She never thought smoking to be a cause for cancer. Later, I found out that a big factor in getting breast cancer was combining smoking with hormone replacement. I didn't get angry at her; I felt bad that it could have been avoided.

Although I do have to say that when I'm taking care of a patient with Alzheimer's or dementia, and I'm being asked the same questions over and over again due to the memory loss, it gets very annoying and frustrating. I have to try to be very patient and understanding. I confess that sometimes it's easier to have patience with the people in the hospital than it is with my own family. And I'm at fault for that.

Barney: No, but I got angry at God a couple of times. When she was in the hospital about two or three weeks, we spent a lot of time talking about what was going to happen. How were we going to handle things? Somewhere in that conversation, and at the same time, we decided that God is good whether she died or not. That changed our lives. From that time on, we didn't feel angry at anyone, just praising God for the nurses because they were doing a great job.

- Was there a silver lining in any of this?

Betty: Good? Maybe a lot of things but not really. My dad and I learned now that we have to do our part to take care of ourselves. Only God has control; let's leave it in His hands. There's so much we can't do. There's a line; beyond that line is God's territory.

Fred: The silver lining was to see how others stepped up and showed genuine Christian compassion and willingness to pray. And to see how close friends showed concern. The silver lining was, my wife and I drew close to the Lord and experienced His presence in tangible ways. It was a great blessing to have the elders of the church gather around both of us and anoint my wife with oil and pray over us. This happened a couple of times.

Wilma: She quit smoking. We were in the surgeon's office, and he recommended a double mastectomy. Mom was still smoking, and the doctor said a plastic surgeon wouldn't touch her to do reconstruction if she didn't stop smoking. Smoking constricts the blood flow so then the incision won't heal. I looked at her and told her to give me her cigarettes. She took them out of her purse and gave them to me. I threw them out—I smashed them. She didn't buy any more, and after that, it was a non-issue.

Also, it sounds odd, but I have a sense of pride that my mom is a breast cancer survivor, three times over. It's a blessing that God spared her.

Barney: Absolutely! We grew a lot closer to each other, and we grew a lot closer to the Lord. As you get older, you look back and see the miracles God has done. Once you get past the problems and get to the other side, it's something you can lean on. You think, "I made it through cancer; this can't be so bad."

- What would you say to encourage someone who has found themselves in the position of caregiver?

Betty: I would look them in their eyes and say, just do one step at a time, like baby steps. Ask God for all the patience you will need because you're going to need a lot. Every day is going to be different. There's going to be good days, so-so days, and worse days. Trust that God is with you, even though you don't see Him.

Fred: Try to live in the moment. Take one day at a time. Don't look too far into the future. Just deal with the tyranny of the urgent, knowing that tomorrow will take care of itself. Focus on the task at hand. Personalize the promises of God that you read in the Bible. Read the Bible daily.

Wilma: My situation was clearly different in terms of being a caregiver. I didn't have a whole lot to do, compared to so many other people. But I would recommend care for the caregiver. They need respite time. They need a day away to take time for themselves and recharge. Sadly, I never offered that to my sister, who was caring for my dying grandmother. I feel bad. My sister got exasperated at us because we never offered help to relieve her or take care of my grandmother—to give my sister a break—and I should have. I look back and I think, *I'm a nurse; I should have done that*, and I didn't. I worked all week doing that [caring for sick people, cleaning, and changing them], and I didn't want to do that on my day off. I know there are places that offer that service. It's definitely necessary for the caregiver going through that. Being unappreciated or not acknowledged for the things we do, it's easy to get embittered.

Barney: It's difficult to advise a caregiver because you don't know what they're going to run into. I would say, don't feel guilty if you can't be everything you need to be. Not everyone is a registered nurse. Do the best you can. You can't feel guilty because it'll make you unhappy and also make the patient unhappy. I would tell a caregiver to never leave anyone in the hospital by themselves. I went back to work after being out for three months, and about 1:00 p.m., my first day back, I got a call from the oncologist, and he said my wife was in the ICU. She had to use the bathroom, and she got up, and she slipped and hit her head, which started bleeding on the brain. With leukemia, your blood gets very thin. You die from bleeding, not leukemia. If I would have been there, she wouldn't have fallen. Another time, when they gave you chemo back then, they would drain some of the chemo out of your line. They put it [the excess chemo] in a cup and left it by her bedside. They meant to dispose of it, but they forgot. Leukemia makes you very thirsty. When my wife woke up, she was thirsty and reached for the cup to drink it, and I was able to stop her. If she drank it, it would have destroyed her esophagus.

I would also tell them, you have to have a lot a patience when they come home. They can't do what they did before. The caregiver has to pick up the slack. And be as encouraging as you can every day. It was during that time that I started a habit, and I still do it to this day. When she gets up in the morning, the first thing she hears is me saying, "Good morning, beautiful lady." When you say something encouraging, it has health benefits. Positive words can help people heal.

RESOURCES FOR CAREGIVERS

Many support groups are willing to come alongside you as you walk through this frightening and often confusing cancer journey. Tim and I personally relied quite heavily on our family, friends, and church. The links provided below are just a smattering of what is available. Services vary from state to state, so don't be afraid to search and contact these organizations to get the help you need. That is the reason they are there.

- The American Cancer Society's website offers a plethora of resources for both the patient and the caregiver, including a helpline telephone number and live-chat feature. https://www.cancer.org/treatment/support-programs-and-services.html
- The Association for Mature American Citizens (AMAC) provides "A Practical To-Do List for Family Caregivers." https://min.amac.us/practical-list-family-caregivers
- Family Caregiver Alliance (FCA) is an advocate to caregivers. Their goal is to improve the quality of life for family caregivers and those who receive their care. https://www.caregiver.org/taking-care-you-self-care-family-caregivers
- USA.gov is the official guide to government information and services and provides helpful tips and information to assist you to care for your loved one. This includes programs for family members of veterans and for those with disabilities

to get paid to render care for their loved one. https://www.usa.gov/disability-caregiver
- The following link, sponsored by the US Department of Health and Human Services, will take you to a site that offers useful advice to those who find themselves in the role of caregiver. https://health.gov/myhealthfinder/topics/everyday-healthy-living/mental-health-and-relationships/get-support-if-you-are-caregiver

EPILOGUE

TEAM CANCER

When I was diagnosed, I didn't want to tell anyone I had cancer. I was determined that this disease wouldn't define me. I adamantly refused to wear pink ribbons. I dug my heels in to avoid being identified with cancer. I didn't want to be a part of the team—but I am. I came to this realization one day during a discussion with Tim about a coworker who just had received his terrifying diagnosis. As the words were leaving my lips, I became aware of just how much my heart ached for this young man. My thoughts also turned to a friend who faced a double mastectomy at the end of the month. I was compelled to fall on my knees and pray for these new members of Team Cancer. That's when it hit me—like it or not, I *am* on the team. It is a part of my history, but because of God's glorious plan for me, I can much better support others and intercede for those in the fight for their lives because I've been there. Now, I can embrace being on Team C. I just have to remember: Christ is the big C!

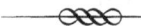

Throughout this book I have spoken to you about my relationship with Jesus Christ. If *you* want to experience the Lord's presence, comfort, power, and wisdom for yourself, it's not hard to do. As you know from what I've written, God loves you so very much and wants you to experience the profound depth of His care. Romans 10:9 promises "that if you confess with your mouth the Lord Jesus and believe in your heart that God has raised Him from the dead, you will be saved."

Simply talk to God and tell Him you are willing to trust Him for salvation. You can tell Him in your own words, or use a simple prayer like this:

> Dear Lord Jesus, I humbly ask You to forgive me of my sins and save me from an eternal separation from God. I know my good works are as filthy rags, and there is nothing I can do to earn salvation. So, by faith, I trust You as Lord and Savior of my life, and I accept Your perfect sacrifice on the cross as sufficient payment for my sins. Through faith in You and You alone, I have eternal life. Thank you for hearing my prayer and loving me unconditionally. Please give me the strength, wisdom, and determination to walk in the center of Your will for my life. In Jesus's name, I pray. Amen.

If you've just prayed this prayer to have your own personal relationship with our wonderful Creator, there's some rejoicing going on in heaven! The Bible says in Luke 15:10, "Likewise, I say to you, there is joy in the presence of the angels of God over one sinner who repents."

If you don't have a Bible, check out the YouVersion Bible at https://www.youversion.com/the-bible-app. This app sends God's Word in 2,062 versions and in 1,372 languages, right to your smartphone or computer. It also has daily devotionals and personal Bible study plans to help you delve into scripture.

In addition, it's really important to connect with other believers. Exercise your faith, and ask God to guide you to a Bible-believing church in your area. Remember, the most important thing to consider when looking for a church is the source of the teaching. Don't worry so much about the style of music or how comfy the chairs are. Everything a church believes should be based on the Bible alone. If a church doesn't believe that the Bible is the inspired Word of God, you should keep looking until you find one that does.

If you have any Christian friends, ask them about the churches they attend, and visit with them. If you do an online search, you can usually listen to virtual sermons. It's also a good idea to see if they have a "What We Believe" or doctrinal statement page to learn more about them.

Thank you for allowing me to share my journey with you. I pray that it is a blessing and that you experience God's gift of shalom, shalom.

> The Lord bless you and keep you;
> The Lord make His face shine upon you,
> And be gracious to you;
> The Lord lift up His countenance upon you,
> And give you peace.
>
> —Numbers 6:24–26

CPSIA information can be obtained
at www.ICGtesting.com
Printed in the USA
JSHW041948270921
19082JS00001B/37